# No Place Like Home?

# Medical Ethics Series
David H. Smith and Robert M. Veatch, Editors

Mary Anderlik, *The Ethics of Managed Care: A Pragmatic Approach*

Norman L. Cantor, *Advance Directives and the Pursuit of Death with Dignity*

Norman L. Cantor, *Legal Frontiers of Death and Dying*

Arthur L. Caplan, *Am I My Brother's Keeper? The Ethical Frontiers of Biomedicine*

Arthur L. Caplan, *If I Were a Rich Man Could I Buy a Pancreas? And Other Essays on the Ethics of Health Care*

James F. Childress, *Practical Reasoning in Bioethics: Principles, Metaphors, and Analogies*

Cynthia B. Cohen, ed., *Casebook on the Termination of Life-Sustaining Treatment and the Care of the Dying*

Cynthia B. Cohen, ed., *New Ways of Making Babies: The Case of Egg Donation*

Roger B. Dworkin, *Limits: The Role of the Law in Bioethical Decision Making*

Larry Gostin, ed., *Surrogate Motherhood: Politics and Privacy*

Christine Grady, *The Search for an AIDS Vaccine: Ethical Issues in the Development and Testing of a Preventive HIV Vaccine*

A Report by the Hastings Center, *Guidelines on the Termination of Life-Sustaining Treatment and the Care of the Dying*

Paul Lauritzen, *Pursuing Parenthood: Ethical Issues in Assisted Reproduction*

Joanne Lynn, M.D., ed., *By No Extraordinary Means: The Choice to Forgo Life-Sustaining Food and Water, Expanded Edition*

William F. May, *The Patient's Ordeal*

Richard W. Momeyer, *Confronting Death*

Thomas H. Murray, Mark A. Rothstein, and Robert F. Murray, Jr. eds., *The Human Genome Project and the Future of Health Care*

Susan B. Rubin, *When Doctors Say No: The Battleground of Medical Futility*

David H. Smith, Kimberly A. Quaid, Roger B. Dworkin, Gregory P. Gramelspacher, Judith A. Granbois, and Gail H. Vance, *Early Warning: Cases and Ethical Guidance for Presymptomatic Testing in Genetic Diseases*

Lois Snyder and Arthur L. Caplan, *Assisted Suicide: Finding Common Ground*

S. Kay Toombs, David Barnard, and Ronald Carson, eds., *Chronic Illness: From Experience to Policy*

Robert M. Veatch, *The Patient as Partner: A Theory of Human-Experimentation Ethics*

Robert M. Veatch, *The Patient-Physician Relation: The Patient as Partner, Part 2*

Leonard Weber, *Business Ethics in Healthcare*

Robert F. Weir, ed., *Physician-Assisted Suicide*

# No Place Like Home?

# Feminist Ethics
## and
## Home
## Health Care

Jennifer A. Parks

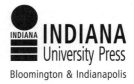

**INDIANA**
University Press
Bloomington & Indianapolis

This book is a publication of

Indiana University Press
601 North Morton Street
Bloomington, Indiana 47404-3797 USA

http://iupress.indiana.edu

*Telephone orders*    800-842-6796
*Fax orders*    812-855-7931
*Orders by e-mail*    iuporder@indiana.edu

The paper used in this publication meets the minimum
requirements of American National Standard for Information
Sciences—Permanence of Paper for Printed Library
Materials, ANSI Z39.48-1984.

Manufactured in the United States of America

**Library of Congress Cataloging-in-Publication Data**

Parks, Jennifer A.
  No place like home? : feminist ethics and home health care / Jennifer
A. Parks.
      p. cm. — (Medical ethics series)
Includes bibliographical references and index.
  ISBN 0-253-34192-2 (alk. paper)
  1. Home health aides—United States. 2. Home care services—United
States. 3. Women in medicine—United States. 4. Feminist ethics.
  [DNLM: 1. Home Care Services—organization & administration. 2.
Feminism. 3. Health Services for the Aged. 4. Home Care
Agencies—organization & administration. 5. Home Health Aides. WY
115 P252n 2003] I. Title. II. Series.
  RA645.35 .P37 2003
    362.1'4—dc21
                                        2002008911
1  2  3  4  5  08  07  06  05  04  03

*For my mother, Lauretta Eva Grace Parks,*
*and my grandmother, Lauretta Abigail Vaughan*

# CONTENTS

*Acknowledgments*                                                    ix

Introduction                                                          1

1. Why Home Care? The Genesis of Home or
   "Community-Based" Care                                             9

2. Examining Philosophies of Home Care                              33

3. Women's Care Work as a Subsidy to the State                      51

4. Caring about the Cared-For                                       73

5. The Personal Is Political: Negotiating Relationships
   within the Home Care Setting                                     92

6. Looking Ahead: Can Home Care Be Reformed?                       120

*Notes*                                                            143
*Works Cited*                                                      153
*Index*                                                            161

# ACKNOWLEDGMENTS

This book could not have been written without the input and support of certain key persons and institutions. I would like to thank Loyola University for funding my summer research in 1999; the paper I wrote that summer went a long way toward developing my thinking on ethics and home health care. I am also grateful to Jim and Hilde Lindemann Nelson and their National Endowment for the Humanities seminar entitled "Bioethics in Particular," which I attended in summer 2000. During this seminar and the time that followed, I developed a great deal of my thinking about identity, relationship, and the value of familial caretaking.

Special acknowledgment must be extended to the staff at Indiana University Press, especially to Marilyn Grobschmidt, who guided me through the publication process. I owe a further debt of gratitude to my colleagues David Ozar and Mark Waymack, who gave me feedback on various ideas contained within this book. My "Topics in Feminism" graduate course in spring 2001 also gave me the opportunity to discuss and debate feminist ethics and caretaking. Thanks to students like Alex de Miranda, Abe Schwab, and Lynn Maitland for their own thoughtful comments on this topic.

It was through edifying relationships with very special women that I found the commitment and stamina to see this project through. As always, Christine Overall and Elisabeth Boetzkes have been mentors, role models, and inspirations. Their ongoing support and affirmation that this was a book worth doing is what helped me to see it through to the end. My mother, Lauretta Parks, provided unfailing love, care, and the "you can do it!" attitude that kept my spirits up throughout the long process.

Most of all, I want to thank my husband and colleague, David Ingram. He had limitless patience with me and my home care obsession; he acted as my sounding board and editor, and most important of all, he helped me to let go of the project when the time came. His terrific sense of humor helped me to keep things in perspective, and his unfailing support showed me what care is all about. For this, and for all his outstanding personal qualities, I am grateful.

# No Place Like Home?

# Introduction

   This book on home care has been a work in progress for almost eleven years. I became interested in writing on the theoretical ethical issues in home care only six years ago, but I had been a home care aide for five years during my graduate education. Indeed, it was as a home care worker, and not as a philosopher, that I learned most about the ethics of home care, for I experienced in the field the best and worst aspects of caretaking. The best aspects involved meeting my clients and building relationships with them; helping them stay in their homes, even if just a little longer; feeling their appreciation for helping them complete simple tasks; and enjoying the sense of being genuinely helpful to others. The worst aspects involved deserting clients when my shifts were over, with them often begging me to stay; my assignment to clients with whom I was not properly trained to work (e.g., clients with quadriplegia, terminal cancer, and severe bedsores); sexual harassment by male clients and physical abuse by clients with dementia (spitting, biting, screaming); my poor remuneration and the gross amount of unpaid, unnoticed labor I performed; and the physical, emotional, and psychological strain that I lived with for that five-year period.

To understand the ethical issues in home care, one must first appreciate what it involves. During my graduate studies—a time of great financial need—economic necessity forced me to take up work outside academia. Given my interest at the time in health care ethics, I saw home care work as an effective way to earn some needed income and be involved in the field. I trained for one week as a home care aide. During this unpaid training, I learned the basics required to assist people in the activities of daily living (ADLs)—bathing, dressing, feeding, changing bandages, transferring clients (e.g., from bed to wheelchair), and lifting—and instrumental activities of daily living (IADLs)—shopping for groceries, preparing meals, doing laundry, and so on. Significantly, at no point did the training staff treat *ethical* issues that we were likely to face in the field. We never discussed the appropriateness of accepting gifts from clients who are often impoverished or suffering dementia, preventing abuse or harassment by clients as well as abuse of clients by caregivers, navigating high-risk situations (e.g., working in dangerous neighborhoods), or the ethics of lying for home care clients. At the time I trained as a home care aide, the focus was on quick training and immediate transition out to the community; there was no time for ethics training and no real appreciation for the ethical issues faced by home care aides.[1]

After training, I began my fieldwork and quickly discovered that no two clients are alike. Some require minimal aid to maintain themselves in their homes: light housekeeping, shopping, laundry, meal preparation. Other clients require more extensive assistance with bathing, dressing, eating, and toileting; and still others are almost completely incapacitated and unable to perform even the simplest of tasks. In some cases, I was sent to clients' homes as a companion, for in many cases the adult children of elderly clients hire attendants to provide comfort and companionship for their aging, isolated, and lonely parents. If clients were temporarily transferred from home to hospital, I was often transferred with them in order to provide extra care that the nursing staff could not (e.g., help with feeding at meal times). If the client's "home" was a nursing facility or psychiatric ward, then that was the venue for my work.

My relationships with the home care supervisors who handled work scheduling was often tenuous at best. By virtue of having control over which clients I was assigned to assist (some being notoriously crotchety or abusive), how many hours I worked, and how much traveling was involved, they wielded a power over me and other home care aides that was often abused. It was understood, for example, that our refusal to accept new clients or fill in at the last minute for aides who called in sick would result in our getting fewer shifts. My supervisors felt free to call at any hour of the day or night to assign work. On one particularly memorable morning, a supervisor began calling at 4 A.M. to request that I make a 5 A.M. shift. She left four messages on my answering machine, demanding that I call the office immediately. (While other health care professionals have this experience of being "on call," there was no sense in which as an aide I was paid to be "on call" twenty-four hours a day for my home care agency. My hourly Canadian wage at the time was $7.15.)

Yet this supervisory abuse of power, such as it is, must also be placed in the context of an exploitative system of care. I never envied the home care supervisors their sometimes Herculean task of trying to find enough aides to cover the required shifts. Indeed, given the high turnover rate in the home health care industry, there is a constant struggle to find enough trained aides who can be sent out to client sites. The case supervisors themselves are overloaded with work. For example, on one day alone I remember a supervisor trying to find workers to cover *twelve* clients.[2] Thus, the ethical issues in home health care arise at the levels of both client site and organization. This book will consider both levels and will often move back and forth between them.

My treatment of the ethics of home care, then, is largely based on my personal experiences. I am assuming, however, that the ethical issues I address and the experiences I relate in this book will resonate with others who are theorists and practitioners in the home care field. I intend to consider home health care through a feminist ethics lens, to address some of the mundane but nevertheless serious ethical issues that arise in the home care setting, to treat the moral perspectives of both caregiver and care recipient in their relationship of care, and to consider broader public policy issues as they relate to the practice of home health care.

I make certain assumptions in this book: first, that home health care is entrenched enough as a mode and venue of care that it is inevitable and cannot be eliminated; second, that individuals invariably prefer home-based over institution-based care; and third, that home care is a feminist issue because its viability as an inexpensive, cost-saving, and effective mode of health care is based on the free and/or cheap care offered by women. I am also assuming that, at best, we can render home health care *minimally* exploitative of women's labor, since the very premise of home care is that "families" (read: women) will offer their free (or cheap) labor out of a sense of obligation.[3] While my ideal system of home health care would be entirely free of exploitation, gender role stereotypes, and gendered expectations of care, I do not hold this out as a realistic vision, given that home care as it has been constructed requires at least some level of exploitation.

From a feminist perspective, empowerment of vulnerable groups is an important aspect of health care provision. Any health care measures that

are implemented should accordingly not serve to uphold harmful stereotypes or further subordinate these groups. A social health policy focusing
on "community-based" care (a misnomer for "home care")[4] must therefore
be examined with concern for the harms and benefits to women and other
vulnerable groups. For example, elderly women, as the largest group receiving home care, cannot be overlooked when considering these harms and
benefits.

As Nora Kizer Bell states, "When one looks closely at the data . . . what
one very quickly discovers is that there are many more elderly women than
there are elderly men" (84). Indeed, statistics indicate that women overwhelmingly outnumber men at the oldest ages such that the provision of
health care for the elderly becomes a women's issue. Since the move toward
home health care disproportionately affects women, it is clearly an issue for
feminist theorists. Yet, as I will argue, home care is a feminist issue for
deeper reasons. Its oppressive structure is significant in itself, since feminists
are concerned with any social structures that detrimentally affect vulnerable groups. Home care is a feminist issue because women have been defined
as caretakers. What matters isn't so much the numbers of female caretakers
but their embeddedness in caring relationships and the gendered burden of
care that impacts women's social, political, economic, and emotional lives.

Some feminist critiques of home care have been damning of the practice.
For instance, sociologist Janet Finch states that nonsexist conceptions of
"community care" are virtually impossible and that it is therefore unre-
formable. Women are so strongly linked to caring and domestic labor, she
argues, that "community care" means little more than care by women.
Given the historical genderedness of caring, Finch argues for the expansion
of institutional care to prevent the exploitation of women. Her feminist critique, however, does not take into account those most seriously affected by
a reversion to institutional care: elderly women.

To be sure, we must realize that elderly women also encounter invisibility in their informal work of caring for their spouses, adult children, and
grandchildren, in doing volunteer work, and in completing the daily tasks
of living. Thus, it is not just younger women as caregivers who are affected
by unrecognized labor; it is also the female elderly. Furthermore, as a recent
article in the *Chicago Tribune* notes, caring for an ailing spouse increases
one's chances of dying by 63 percent due to the strain of providing such
care.[5]

Given the extent to which elderly women outnumber elderly men, it is
clear that care by females will, in most cases, be preferred over care by
males. Elderly women overwhelmingly request female caregivers; the personal nature of the care required tends to make these vulnerable elderly

women uncomfortable with male assistance with their ADLs. The power differential between elderly women and younger men is also a concern: By being placed under care by males, elderly women may be put at risk (or, at least, perceive themselves at risk). Thus, contrary to Finch's claim, there *is* a nonsexist basis for the widespread preference for female caretakers in home health care.[6]

It seems that feminists are trapped by incommensurable commitments: (1) providing care to dependents (elderly women in particular) who choose to be cared for at home by women; (2) petitioning for a shift to institution-based care (such as nursing homes); or (3) refusing to maintain the gendered burden of care in any of its manifestations. As I will argue in the chapters that follow, women should not cease their current provision of care. As long as women constitute the greatest portion of elderly care recipients who desire female caregiving, and as long as there are women who are willing to provide the required care despite the low pay, home health care is justified. But as a society we must simultaneously petition for justice in terms of fairness, the equal distribution of care work between men and women, and economic justice.

In addition, on the social level, we must reconsider the ethic that undergirds the practice of home health care, for as I will also argue in this book, the autonomy-based ethic that guides acute care cannot satisfactorily address the ethical issues that arise for caregivers and care receivers in the home care setting. For instance, the decision concerning a client's continued care in the home is not satisfactorily made by a straightforward appeal to her autonomy,[7] for the client is not the only subject of concern. The caretakers, family members, and other citizens living in close proximity to the home care client are also integral to the decision. If the client is leaving burners on in her apartment, for example, then she is clearly putting the other residents of her apartment complex in danger. Thus, rather than taking a traditional autonomy-based approach to home health care, I will argue for a feminist "relational autonomy" model. This approach does not invoke the traditional principle of autonomy to which bioethicists so commonly appeal; rather, it conceives of autonomy as resulting from relationships of care and concern. On this view, autonomy develops *because of,* not in spite of, our relationships with others. So while I argue that a conception of autonomy should be maintained, it must be radically reconceived in response to these feminist critiques. The traditional conception of autonomy is false and misleading, since we are born into a network of relationships and our self-understandings and life plans are continuously modified within this context throughout our lives. Indeed, as I hope to convince my readers, the traditional concept of autonomy as independence and self-sufficiency has limited value in resolving ethical issues in home health care and other long-term care settings.[8]

I begin by analyzing the genesis of home or "community-based" care. In order to explore the ethics of home health care, we must first consider its origins. As hospitals discharge patients "sicker and quicker," as the population ages, as the cost of nursing home care continues to rise, and as people value care within the privacy and comfort of their own abodes, home health care becomes an increasingly desirable mode of caregiving. Furthermore, since the care of prematurely discharged elderly patients falls largely on female family members, and the remaining inadequate allotment of government-funded care is carried out by poorly paid, nonprofessional home care aides, the cost savings of home-based care may prove great.

After considering its economic rationale, I will examine the sometimes warring philosophies behind the practice of home care. Chapter 2 will address the central values expressed in the very structure and delivery of home care services. Those central values—rooted in the market-driven, managed care model of care provision—go to the core of what home care stands for, the purpose it is meant to serve, and the individuals to whom it applies. At the same time, home care practitioners express a noncommercial ethic that comes out of their work with real persons.

Chapter 3 will explore the ethics of home health care from a feminist perspective. Such a feminist ethical critique of home care is called for, given the spread of the practice and the very small number of feminists who have taken up the *ethical* issues in this system of care.[9] I will focus on the way in which home health care perverts the feminist ethic of care to naturalize women's caring and co-opt their care work, and consider the requirements for an ethic rich enough to guide home care. As I will argue, feminists must go beyond an "ethic of care" to consider the requirements of justice for home care aides and unpaid or poorly paid female family members. So, as I will argue, feminist moral theorists like Nel Noddings (1984) should be read critically for their failure to take seriously the requirements of justice in provisions of care. Following feminist philosopher Eva Kittay's 1999 critique of dependency work and dependency workers, I will argue that home caregiving must be included as one of the social institutions that is subjected to the demands for justice.

However, as chapter 4 will indicate, feminist ethicists must concern themselves with justice not only for caregivers but also for care recipients. Feminist critiques of domination and subordination within health care systems caution us not to objectify and further subordinate recipients of care, for persons dependent on care from others are moral agents that are deserving of equal moral consideration. In addition, since many home care recipients are elderly women, we must attend to their call for justice and recognition in a way that balances caretakers' needs. As Jay Arbor and Sara Ginn have indicated, feminism has a history of focusing on younger women's issues to the detriment of our elders; in the area of home health care, we cannot afford this oversight.

My further purpose in chapter 4 is to consider the effectiveness of *relational autonomy* in negotiating home care relationships. Following my critique of traditional conceptions of autonomy, I will argue that we need to fundamentally reconceive ourselves as independent, autonomous, rational, and self-sufficient to understand them as socially embedded, bound by particular others in relationships of dependency, care, and concern.

Chapter 5 will consider a variety of relationships and ethical questions that arise within the home care setting in order to ponder the sometimes mundane (but nonetheless pressing) ethical dilemmas associated with home care. One of the trenchant problems in this practice is how to negotiate relationships within the home setting. To this end I will treat issues like the appropriateness of accepting gifts from clients, racism in home care relationships, removing clients from their homes, and paid family caretaking. As I will argue, these issues are connected by a general concern with the self in relationship to others.

The final chapter will consider ways in which home care can be reformed to make it a morally better practice. My concern will be with making home care better for clients and better for caretakers—especially those frontline workers who are the lowest paid and least respected. I will argue that we need to take health care out of a market system in order to reform home care as a practice. Since the two are closely connected, we cannot hope for real change in the home care sector if we don't address the macro problems with our current system of health care. Applying Marxist and feminist critiques, I will argue that our current system of home care is exploitative and alienating and that it devalues the work *as* work. In order to address the needs of clients and caretakers, we need to effect change in home care, and as I will argue, this change is already slowly taking place through the move to unionize home care workers.

There are some points to keep in mind concerning my use of terminology in this book. First of all, readers should note my use of the term *caretaking* rather than *caregiving*. I employ this term to remind my audience that care should not be viewed as merely a "gift" to be given by women but that it is, indeed, work. By employing this less common term, I hope to keep readers mindful of the way we commonly think about care work and to encourage resistance to such traditional conceptions of it.

Second, though I struggled with my terminology with reference to care recipients, I settled on the common practice in home health care of calling them *clients*. While this term smacks of a certain social contractarianism (where "clients" contract with caretakers to receive care), it nevertheless preserves the agency of individuals who receive home care services. For this reason, and for lack of a better term, I will adopt this more common usage.

Third, readers should be conscious of my appeal to the "public" and "private" spheres. Wherever these terms appear in this book, they should be read in scare quotes, though for the sake of keeping my text clean, I will not use scare quotes every time they appear. I intend the terms to be used self-consciously, with full awareness of the ways in which the so-called public and private spheres overlap. The conception of these spheres as separate and distinct does violence to our actual life experiences. As John Stuart Mill indicates, it is not always possible to distinguish between "private" acts that concern only myself—acts that do not harm the interests of others—and "public" ones.

Finally, a note about my use of the terms *home health care* and *home care*. While some theorists distinguish these terms from one another, I will use them interchangeably. Whether clients require home services for serious health problems or merely for help with their ADLs and IADLs, they usually require the assistance of home care aides. To avoid repetition of the same term throughout the book, then, I will use *home care* and *home health care* to denote the practice of providing care at home to persons with dependency needs.

I intend this book to be used as a resource for philosophy, women's studies, political science, and nursing courses. My purpose is to treat home health care as just one particular example of how women's care work is exploited by the state. I see this exploitation, however, as binding home care to other forms of caregiving (child care, nursing home care, care for people with disabilities). My call to respond to women's caretaking in home care should be extended to these other areas where caretakers are poorly remunerated and highly exploited.

# 1 Why Home Care?

## The Genesis of Home or "Community-Based" Care

The answer to the question "Why home health care?" involves a panoply of considerations. This chapter will treat the rising popularity of home care, that is, the circumstances that have led to its ascendancy through the 1980s and 1990s, and what I see as the largely exploitative bases for its practice. Throughout this chapter and the rest of the book, I will treat home health care as an enterprise of deep ethical import, for bound up with its practice are questions about how we value human relationships (and which relationships we value), what counts as work (and who gets to decide), the worth of caretaking, and the kind of system through which we can best provide services to some of the most vulnerable members of our communities.

This chapter will develop my thesis that home health care, as practiced within the current social and political climate, is riddled with ethical problems. Currently, home care is carried out on the assumption that women will either do the caretaking for free (as daughters, granddaughters, daughters-in-law, sisters, spouses, lovers, and neighbors) or for minimum wage.

To be sure, home health care providers in the United States (that is, the companies that are responsible for providing care for clients) are hamstrung by the broader system of health care, of which home health is only a part. Providers complain that the high cost of health care in the United States, coupled with the limits on reimbursement by Medicare and private insurers, means that it is difficult to stay afloat or provide services effectively to clients who are in need of them. Thus, some of the ethical problems associated with the delivery of home health care start at the macro level, where one finds a system of managed care that sets the stage for the practice of home health care.

Ultimately, as I will argue, the United States requires an expanded government role in overseeing home care. While as a feminist I am not entirely comfortable with the capacity for the state to combat egregious social injustices, there is little hope for a fair system of home health care delivery if the state is not involved at a basic level. And while some critics have recommended a system of *managed* home health care that is based on the broader managed health care system, in chapter 3 I will argue that such an approach overlooks some of the most trenchant problems associated with this type of care. From the feminist perspective for which I am advocating, we need to view and appreciate care done in the home for what it is: a subsidy provided by women to the state.[1] Once we take seriously the notion that the *state* and not just the individual family benefits from the formal and informal care work done by women, then we can begin to ask questions like that posed by Martha Fineman: "Is it fair that the market and the state (which are totally dependent on caretaking labor and in no way self-sufficient or independent from caretaking) escape responsibility for dependency and continue to be freeloaders (or free riders) on the backs of caretakers and families?" (25).

First, in order to answer the question "why home health care?" let us consider the system in its current manifestation: how we inherited the present mode of delivery, how it works, and how it is overseen. Then in chapter 3 I will apply a feminist lens to argue the need for a socialized system of home care. This system would provide both formal and informal caretakers with support in the form of payment, subsidies, paid family leaves, and income tax breaks.

### Home Care as "Homecoming"

While home care is often heralded as a "new" care paradigm, the practice is not new. On the contrary, it is a return to ways of providing for the ill and frail that have a long history, both in the United States and abroad.

Thus, the de-institutionalization movement—the glorifying of home or "community-based" care as the answer to hospital or nursing home care—is a "homecoming" in more than one sense of the word. While patients are, indeed, coming home sooner, home care is also a return to a way of care-taking that is part of our social history. Yet this hearkening back to com-munal ways of caring for needy citizens is also a hearkening back to certain gendered care expectations that, in a feminist age, are far more difficult to justify.

One assumption behind the de-institutionalization movement is that the United States can no longer afford the high costs of institution-based care. Thus one finds the broad appeal of home health services, where individuals can be discharged from expensive care institutions in order to receive cheap-er, intermittent, at-home care. The answer to the question "Why home health care?" then is in part economic because, at least initially, home care was seen as a much cheaper option, with huge potential savings over institution-based care.[2]

A second assumption behind the move to "community" care is that most patients would prefer to receive treatment and recuperate in the com-fort of their own homes. This assumption may not be far off, for as Martha Holstein has averred,

> Caregiving is essential if older people with mental or physical disabilities are to remain at home, where they clearly want to be, especially given the options available. Visit any nursing home and you will find that even pa-tients seriously affected by dementing illnesses plead for home. Home has powerful emotional and symbolic meanings. It connotes family, security, comfort, treasured memories, and even "independence." If one is home, then one is not fully "sick." Implicit norms about independence, auton-omy, and productivity reinforce the lure of home (228).

Thus, the ideological bases for home health care are both economic and symbolic. They are economic in that home care is a supposedly cheaper op-tion that will ideally result in cuts to health care spending. And they are symbolic in that home care symbolizes all the positive associations we have with hearth and home. Whether or not patients are *actually* better off in their own homes (that is safer, more comfortable, more secure, better cared-for), home care symbolizes a "kinder, gentler" form of health care delivery where patients can remain in the bosoms of their families.

The economic justification for home health care is intricately tied to the United States health care system as it is currently run. At the macro level, since the late 1970s and early 1980s, health care in the United States has gone through market reform. This reform has resulted in a shift from fee-

for-service payment for health care (where physicians had the freedom to
charge as they saw fit for health care services) to managed care, where
health maintenance organizations (HMOs) act as third-party payers to
physicians, placing caps on the fees that physicians are entitled to charge.
In the early 1980s, a system of managed care was hailed as the answer to
the problem of gross inflation of health care costs. For example, during the
Reagan administration, costs for health care services ballooned at a rate of
20 percent per year (Kuttner, 1997), in part because of the rise of third-
party payers, where physicians were no longer directly billing individual patients for their health care. While the pre-insurance era kept health care
costs down because physicians were reluctant to overcharge their often
poor or financially strapped patients, the rise of health insurance meant that
they could bill insurance companies at much higher rates without bank-
rupting individual families. Yet because health care insurance was by this
time employment-based, employers found the rising costs of insuring workers impossible to bear. Employers could not afford this type of cost inflation, and they looked for other ways of providing health care to their
employees. New health insurance provision came in the form of managed
care organizations, which promised to ratchet down employers' insurance
costs by focusing on good preventive care for employees. By the mid-1980s,
health care reform had taken place as market reform. An important aspect
of such change was the free-market takeover of health care by way of corporate mergers and the rise of the HMO.

The aims of managed care are honorable: to lower and control health
care costs in order to provide coverage that is comprehensive and maximally inclusive. Since the gross inflation of health care costs was caused by
a host of problems such as duplication of services, overprescribing of medications for patients, and the ordering of unnecessary testing, managed care
also purported to best serve patients, since overmedication and unnecessary
testing put them at needless medical risk.

But the advent of managed care was not the panacea that was promised.
Since the coming of managed care to America, the focus has not been pa-
tient-centered but rather commerce-centered; that is, managed care organizations are part of the free market, run on a for-profit basis. This means
that the goals of health care have concerned not patients' ends but corporate ends of fiscal viability and profitability. Furthermore, since health care
insurance continues to be employment-based, managed care is not maximally inclusive. On the contrary, close to 45 million Americans are unin-
sured or underinsured.[3] Since health care continues to be carried out in the
marketplace on a for-profit basis, and since HMOs have swiftly become the
modus operandi in health care, it has become difficult to effectively argue

for any other system of health care. And where health care is marketized, it is inevitable that branches of health care—such as home care and nursing home care—will follow suit.

Many home care theorists and commentators assume the managed care model for the provision of home care services. For example, Kathryn Christiansen sees a managed home care model as inevitable:

> Clearly the macro-level health care paradigm has changed, and the home care field must respond accordingly. Managed care is fast becoming the new home care paradigm, and with it comes a new set of rules. With new rules come new opportunities. (14–15)

In what follows, I will describe what home care currently looks like within the U.S. system of managed care. I hope to indicate the serious shortcomings of such a system and the ways in which the system is unjustly founded on women's free, and cheap, labor.

### Home Care as Managed Care

In the midst of sweeping health care change at the macro level, the cottage industry of home health care came onto the scene in the early 1980s. But this "cottage industry" quickly became a core service rather than an extra service to meet the needs of a specific group of patients. And the idea that home care could be an effective and economical form of caretaking was not limited to the United States. In Canada, for example, the Ontario Ministry of Health announced in 1992 that it would try to reduce health care costs by moving health care out of the hospital and back into the community. In the United States, "the market for home care services grew from $6.1 billion in 1986 to $11.1 billion in 1991" (Linne, 5), and the demand has continued to grow.

But the flourishing of home care in the United States has occurred within the system of managed care that I have outlined, and this macro system has directly influenced the direction that home care has taken. For example, home care is largely run on a for-profit basis, with individual home care providers competing for clients and contracts. And within the broader system of managed care, providers face restrictions on services for which they can bill and Medicare caps that often leave them caring without remuneration for clients.

The advent of Diagnosis Related Groups (DRGs) that were encoded by 1983 federal law has also impacted home care services, as it resulted in an increased demand for such services due to reduced hospital stays for many patients. DRGs is a system established by the federal government that sets, for all Medicare patients and for each possible diagnosis, an average length of hospital stay and cost of in-patient treatment. Under the DRG system, hospitals are paid prospectively the established amount for each patient with a given diagnosis, regardless of the actual cost of treatment. This prospective payment system has resulted in hospitals discharging patients earlier than in the past; a good number of these patients require follow-up care, and here home health providers have been key. Yet limits set by DRGs also impact home health providers such that reimbursement for services may cease before a client is truly capable of managing on her own; in such cases, providers are in a position to continue services without being paid. Providers must continue services without being paid because the law stipulates that home care agencies cannot just "drop" patients without providing for an equivalent or more appropriate setting.

### Medicare, Medicaid, and Home Care

Medicare and Medicaid play a central role in the provision of home care services. Since a vast number of home care recipients are over age 65, and Medicare was put in place to provide health insurance for elderly citizens, the growth of the home care industry has resulted in a huge burden on Medicare. For example, Medicare expenditures on home health care (both personal and skilled care services) skyrocketed from "just under $4 billion in 1990 to more than $18 billion in 1996" (Feder et al., 44).

Medicare sets limits on reimbursable care that places home care providers in an even more precarious position. For example, to be eligible for reimbursed home care services under the Medicare plan, patients must meet the following requirements: The patient must be homebound—that is, he or she must have a physical or medical condition that prevents him or her from going out (except for medical appointments), and the patient must require skilled and intermittent care. This means that if the patient does not constantly require the skilled services of a medical professional (i.e., nursing, physical therapy, or speech therapy), then he or she is not eligible for any other kinds of home care service, including occupational therapy or the essential home aide services. Also, patients must have a referring physician who has approved the plan of treatment and identified the patient's skilled need. This means that every two months physicians must approve the services, frequency, and duration of care that is to be provided.

The result is that, under the current free market model, home care providers may refuse services to home care clients if the services are not reimbursed by Medicare; indeed, providers may choose not to take on clients at all because of the likely costs involved to the provider itself. And the result is that many clients who require home care services—but who do not meet the "skilled needs" requirement—are left to struggle on their own or with the assistance of unpaid family caretakers if they are available.

A war of sorts has been waged between Medicare and Medicaid over coverage for home care services. Medicare is a federally funded program that finances health care for elderly citizens; Medicaid is a largely state-run health insurance program for the poorest U.S. citizens. Under Medicaid policy each state shares with the federal government financial responsibility for health care services. Yet the policies of these two programs seem less focused on citizens' care needs and more concerned with shifting responsibility from one to the other. Within a context where there is a paucity of long-term care policies, this shifting of responsibility has resulted in a lack of appropriate care for those most in need.

Medicaid (the federal/state program), which provides health insurance for citizens who fall below the level of subsistence, is the primary financier of long-term care services in the United States.[4] Medicaid is in place to finance care for both the poor and those who are rendered poor after spending their assets on medical or long-term care. As some theorists point out,

> Federal rules entitle elderly and disabled persons to Medicaid benefits if their incomes and assets are low enough to qualify them for the federal Supplemental Security Income (SSI) cash assistance program—in 2000, income of no more than $532 per month, and nonhousing assets less than or equal to $2,000 for individuals. Most states allow people to become eligible under "medically needy" provisions if they spend down their income and assets on care. (Feder et al., 43)

Medicaid, unlike Medicare, allows coverage for personal at-home services regardless of whether a patient requires skilled care services.

Because Medicaid is not just federally but also state funded, one finds large variations in long-term care spending across the states. For example, in 1998, Medicaid spending ranged from $120 per resident in some states to more than three times that amount in others. Some states limit the number of persons enrolled in their programs, despite the supposed general applicability of federal requirements. Both home care and nursing home care are targets for Medicaid cuts, since these two forms of long-term care constitute the lion's share of long-term care spending.

By contrast, Medicare spending on home care services has ballooned and fallen since the late 1980s such that between 1982 and 1994 the number of people receiving Medicare-funded assistance rose from 4 percent to 10 percent (Feder et al., 45). But again, since the mid-1990s, Medicare has been cutting back on assistance for home care services as a direct result of the 1997 Balanced Budget Act (BBA). By 1999, Medicare had cut spending on services by 45 percent, to less than $10 billion.[5]

This ebb and flow in home care spending is related to the lack of policy surrounding Medicaid and Medicare coverage of long-term care services. For example, no *explicit* policy has been formulated surrounding the provision of home care services. The expansion of Medicare home health coverage occurred without discussion of the roles that Medicaid, Medicare, private insurance, and out-of-pocket coverage should play. As a result, we don't know whether Medicare home care benefits are allocated fairly (since it covers skilled home health needs but not personal care needs) and whether it is carried out efficiently (with its heavy reliance on home care agencies).

As I will argue in chapter 6, Amartya Sen's capabilities model may better address the needs of persons receiving home care benefits. Sen argues that a decent system of distribution should ensure that basic human capabilities are realized. By "capabilities," Sen means promoting the kinds of human flourishing, function, and abilities that are an important part of our common public life. Current home care dialogue focuses on monetary allotments and ignores the development or support of human capabilities (like holding a job, fulfilling educational goals, receiving decent care). Since you cannot buy capabilities, addressing the economics of home care provision fails to achieve this important good. By focusing on Medicare/Medicaid provision, we emphasize medical needs and fail to address our social ones.

The absence of clear long-term care policy points to another serious problem: a lack of consensus concerning the norms governing home care. While I will treat this issue in detail in chapter 2, it is worth noting here that home care is being practiced absent any clear sense of the norms and values that support it. As a result, the fallback norm in practice is one that encourages agencies to limit spending on services, resulting in a paucity of care for most citizens except the very wealthiest.

When considering how home care is funded, one cannot overlook the role played by private insurance and out-of-pocket spending. While Medicare and Medicaid represent some of the largest financiers of home care services, individual patients and their families spend a considerable amount.

### Private Insurance and Out-of-Pocket Spending

Private insurance finances approximately 7 percent of long-term care coverage and so does not represent a large insurance pool. What I am here calling "private insurance" for home care services is constituted by either private health insurance coverage or the recently available long-term care insurance. Some private health care plans include limited home care coverage, but this coverage is usually short-term and follows a patient's discharge from hospital. Private health insurers have been unwilling to cover the high cost of home care services that attend to the activities of daily living (ADLs) and instrumental activities of daily living (IADLs) of dependent insurees, since the costs associated with meeting patients' nonskilled needs can be astronomical. As a result, one finds the advent of long-term care insurance.

This type of private insurance is a response to the lack of coverage available for home care services. The purpose of long-term care insurance is to cover the costs associated with home care services and to provide individuals and families with extended coverage that will meet their home health care needs. Given the fragmentary nature of coverage for home care services, and the requirement that an individual or family must "spend down" all assets in order to be eligible for state insurance programs like Medicaid, long-term care insurance is a new cottage industry. But this type of insurance has not yet caught on, since "as of the end of 1996 fewer than five million policies had been sold" (Feder et al., 42).

More significant is the out-of-pocket familial spending on home care services necessitated by the abysmal financial structure surrounding it. In 1998, the use of private financial resources to pay for nursing home and home health costs constituted 26 percent of funding for long-term care (Feder et al., 41). In the absence of an insurance system (both public and private) that spreads across the population the financial risk associated with home care, individuals and/or families are paying out-of-pocket to meet their care needs. And given the costs involved with home care services, families who are forced to pay for them face unacceptable financial risks.

As I will indicate in chapter 3, financial risks are not the only kinds of perils facing patients who pay out-of-pocket. In addition to financial burdens, family members are required to reduce their work hours, retire early, or quit their jobs in order to perform familial caretaking tasks for at-home patients. The impact of these solutions on the economic stability, career paths, morale, and even physical health of caretakers and their families can be serious. For example, as one study of elderly caretakers indicates:

> The strain of caring for an ailing husband or wife can be deadly for the elderly. Researchers found that elderly spouses who are strained by providing such care were 63 percent more likely to die during the four-year period of their study. . . . Stephen McConnell, vice president for public policy at the Alzheimer's Association, said the study underscores the need to

support caregivers. He noted that Medicare covers elderly caregivers if they get sick but does not pay for help that could keep them from falling ill.[6]

One of the grave problems with home care policy is the way in which our collective responsibility for the health of all our citizens is delegated to the private sphere of the family. By failing to take up our collective responsibility, we fail one another in tangible, serious ways. We allow individuals and families to be bankrupted, torn apart, and physically and emotionally traumatized by the burden of care.

Thus far I have argued that home health care is premised on a system of managed care that focuses on limiting care and cutting costs. It is characterized by shifting, unstable, and sometimes irrational care plans. Absent any clear-cut policies on the provision of long-term care services, the fallback norm in home care service provision has been to limit costs by limiting care. If home care *is* a cheaper, more viable option than institution-based care, then it is only because care services have been so severely restricted. The severe restrictions on home care services mean that patients and their families (if they have them) make up the difference by performing caretaking on an informal basis and by providing out-of-pocket funding for their care needs.

Familial caretaking plays a monumental role in the provision of home care; furthermore, the very fiscal viability of home care is premised on the free labor provided by patients' families. In what follows, I will indicate how familial caretaking results in cost-saving for the state; I will also show that threading through the practice of home care is the assumption that family members are the natural caretakers.

### Familial Caretaking: The Hidden Home Care Resource

Much has been written to date on issues surrounding familial caretaking. These writings come from a variety of disciplines and perspectives, including feminism, philosophy, sociology, anthropology, law, and medicine.[7] In considering the role of informal care in home care delivery, I will draw upon these resources to indicate the deep connection between home care and the family unit. Without families, home care simply cannot meet society's caretaking needs. The trope of the family as stable, loving, altruistic, and highly functional serves the practice of home care, for it is by drawing on such tropes that family members are recruited to serve the state. Of course, such service is never perceived as service to the state, since care for our loved ones is supposed to spring spontaneously and altruistically from our genetic and social ties with them. But the free labor provided by families *is* a social service that results in savings for the state; I will pursue this claim in chapter 3 by arguing for a system that recognizes and remunerates this care work. First, however, let us consider how "voluntary" familial care work fits within our current system of home care service.

Much of the support for home care services comes from out-of-pocket expenditures by patients and/or their families. But there is a figure that is absent in all these calculations of expenditures on home care services: the cost savings to the state that is part of familial caretaking and the costs absorbed by individual families in order to provide the care. One study, for example, estimates that the economic value of informal caretaking in the United States was $196 billion in 1997. This figure is more than formal home health care services and nursing home care, which together cost approximately $115 billion. To say that familial caretaking represents government savings is therefore a massive understatement (Arno et al.).

The caretaking done by (mostly female) family members falls outside the market economy and is not socially and politically visible, since it takes place in the "private sphere" of the home. As a result, the economic value of this work is largely unrecognized, though ironically its value is assumed within the structure and delivery of home care services. Consider an example to understand how familial caretaking is taken for granted within the home care system.

Maxwell Walsh is an 84-year-old man who was recently hospitalized after a serious car accident. As his wife, Shirley, was backing out of a parking space, she knocked Maxwell over with the open car door. He suffered broken ribs, contusions, and a serious concussion and spent several weeks in a hospital. Due to his physical injuries, serious weight loss, and weakening from lying in bed, his ability to walk, even with a walker, was seriously compromised. Toward the end of his hospital stay, Maxwell began physical and occupational therapy. Shirley visited him regularly, as did his son and daughter-in-law. His other son and daughter visited when possible, but they lived out of state, so regular visits were difficult.

As part of discharge planning, Maxwell's physician referred him to home health services. Through Medicare benefits, and because Maxwell had skilled care needs (requiring physical and occupational therapy), Maxwell and Shirley were able to secure some home care services for the first six weeks. However, the hours allocated were few: Maxwell received three two-hour therapy sessions per week for the first four weeks; then hours were cut to two two-hour sessions per week. There was no time allotment for home health aide services to help Maxwell with his ADLs or IADLs.

Shirley Walsh is 79 years old. She lives with Maxwell in their mobile home community. Before Maxwell's discharge from the hospital, she came down with pneumonia, which left her weak, exhausted, and irritable. Shirley was not ready for her husband's return, as she could hardly meet her own needs. And his care needs were, indeed, complex, as he had a very weak heart and prostate cancer in addition to his injuries from the accident. Physically weak, he wet his bed every night. Shirley had to change his sheets and do laundry daily.

The only relief to Shirley came in the form of her son and daughter-in-law, who lived thirty minutes away and came regularly to help care for Maxwell. But much of the time Shirley was left alone with Maxwell; she worried that she could not continue to meet his care needs. In addition, Maxwell proved to be uncooperative with her when they were alone, refusing to use his walker as he was instructed by his home care supervisor and sometimes falling as a result. Shirley knew that one of these falls could seriously hurt Maxwell and that she should press the issue with their home care provider. But she also knew that if she refused to continue caring at home for Maxwell, he would be sent to a long-term care facility. Shirley didn't want to see her husband back in one of "those places," where he was mostly left in bed and where he got little exercise or stimulation.

Their situation is typical of how home care services are allotted. Given the restrictions placed on Medicare reimbursement for home care, the expectation is that family members will "supplement" the care hours offered by home care providers. But as we can see in the case of Maxwell and Shirley Walsh, the "supplementing" comes from the home care agency, not the family. Families fulfill most of the care requirements with home care services filling in clients' skilled care needs.

Martha Holstein indicates how caretaking is accomplished within the familial unit. She claims that women constitute 70 percent of all caretakers and 77 percent of children giving care. Furthermore, she claims,

> Almost one-third of all caregivers of frail elderly persons are adult daughters; while sons also provide care, they generally assume instrumental and time-flexible tasks like paying bills or mowing the lawn. Daughters shoulder tasks that keep them on call 24 hours a day, with little or no assistance, while sons typically get help from their wives. Paid services may also be distributed unequally—men caring for elderly spouses or parents seem to obtain more paid in-home services than their female counterparts. . . . In practice, daughters reduce work, while men reduce caregiving, and as a result, daughters are more likely than sons to perceive caregiving as stressful. (230)

The stresses of caretaking devolve upon families, but as Holstein points out, "family" is a euphemism for care by women (as is the notion of "community-based" care).

I attribute the heavy reliance by the home care industry on familial caretaking to two important historical developments: first, the traditional completion of care work by women within the private sphere; and second, the paradigm of acute care that generally governs medicine in the United States. In what follows I will develop these points to indicate why families are so central to the practice of home health care.

### Women as Caretakers

Feminist attention has focused on women as primary caretakers in situations of community care. Janet Finch, like many other feminist critics of community care,[8] focuses on the way in which expansion of community care services results in a regression of women's rights and interests. The broad interest in expanding community care is, she argues, based on the assumption that women will assume these caring roles on either a volunteer basis or for extremely low pay. The entire structure of community care, therefore, relies on an oppressive historical model of women as homemakers and caretakers in the private sphere of the home. "Family care" of elderly people is euphemistic for care of the elderly by women; thus, "'community' care for the elderly . . . depends primarily on the ability and willingness of women to provide that care" (Finch, 16).

Caring is tied not only to women but to the private sphere where intimate relationships flourish. This is primarily the sphere of the home and family. Since women have been linked historically to the private sphere of the home, the task of caring again comes full circle to an association with women. And women internalize this association with caring such that feelings of guilt arise if they are charged with not caring enough or, worse, not caring at all.

Women's caring labor has been rendered invisible since the industrial revolution. Prior to industrialization, in the "Old Order," the skills contributed by women were indispensable to survival. As Barbara Ehrenreich and Deirdre English state, "All women were expected to have learned, from their mothers and grandmothers, the skills of raising children, healing common illnesses, healing the sick." Following industrialization, however, this indispensable work in the home ceased to be acknowledged (and thus effectively ceased to exist) when the public and private realms were split apart. As these authors suggest, "The womanly skills which the economy of the Old Order had depended on have been torn away—removing what had been the source of women's dignity in even the most oppressive circumstances" (8–9, 11).

In the current context, this identification of women with their caring role and responsibilities is a serious issue for feminist critics. According to

Finch, there are no nonsexist alternatives to community care because all such notions depend upon the use of women and their free (or cheap) labor. Finch therefore concludes that, with regard to social policy, we must move away from the community care model and concentrate on improving and expanding institutional care.

Women bear the burden of home care's poorly remunerated formal labor and its unremunerated informal labor. Some critics therefore assert that home care represents a regression of women's interests because it takes us back to the public/private distinction where women work in the private realm of the home and where men have a "real" job outside of the home. Hilary Graham asserts, "Caring tends to be associated not only with women, but with those private places where intimate relations with women are found. Specifically, caring is associated with the home and family" (16). Finch agrees, arguing that there are powerful associations of women with caring such that nonsexist forms of community care are impossible without a cultural revolution.

Chapter 3 will expand on this issue of justice and women's care work; for my purposes here, it is enough to acknowledge the gendered history of caretaking in order to see how this history feeds into the expectation that women will complete care tasks for their elderly and ill loved ones.

The family is a core unit of home care services for another important historical reason: Health care has been structured around an acute care paradigm such that chronic care needs are not met within the system. Ironically, this means that even home care services—which are premised on patients' chronic, long-term care needs—are carried out based on an acute care model. For example, one can only receive home care services through Medicare if the services immediately follow discharge from a hospital, so in this way even home care services are premised on an acute care paradigm. This ironically renders those who do not experience an acute medical situation without recourse, since their medical situations are not "acute" enough to qualify them for chronic care services!

### On the Paradigm of Acute Care and the Myth of Self-Control

The language of control is used so freely within medical and social discourse and is so integral to our culture that it leads to our cultural fixation on controllable acute medical emergencies. Indeed, as many authors have noted, although chronic illness is a primary health problem in North America, especially among the aged, our health care model remains focused on acute care emergencies.[9] As a result, chronic and palliative care are not satisfactorily represented in medicine because such models of care admit to the reality of human aging, disability, illness, and our lack of control over our health and our bodies. Current medical practice—and the focus on acute care measures—thus conceals the extent to which many individuals live with chronic health problems and/or disability.

Acute care is characterized by the high-tech monitoring of acute illnesses, complex diagnostic procedures, and treatable conditions: The medical problem is definable, recognized (both socially and medically), and controllable at the acute stage. Victims in acute care situations (car accident victims, for example) present medical problems that are immediately recognizable and treatable: internal bleeding, cracked ribs, punctured lungs, and so on. Chronic care, by contrast, is characterized by uncertainty of problem and outcome, no social and often no medical recognition of the problem (migraines of unknown origin, for example), and lack of control.

It is the very possibility of treatment, diagnosis, and control in acute medical situations that leads to our paradigm of acute care. This care paradigm supports the social emphasis we place upon control, health, and personal autonomy. As Susan Wendell claims, "Modern Western medicine plays into and conforms to our cultural myth that the body can be controlled. . . . Surgery and saving lives bolster the illusion of control much better than does the long, patient process of rehabilitation or the management of long-term illness" (72). Thus, our health care system focuses on acute care, given the possibilities in acute medical treatment for saving lives, curing illnesses, and maintaining the false illusion of control that is so important to our culture. The main goal of medicine thus comes to be, as it is in wider society, to control the body. This is not often possible in chronic care situations, and it is worse in palliative care where the goal is to ease individuals into death. Since these care models admit to the frailty of the human body and life in general, they fail as medical paradigms, despite the large number of individuals who are (or will be) chronically ill, disabled, or dying.

Acute care is also paradigmatic because of the autonomous self it presupposes, that is, one that is free from external limits or constraints, including bodily ones.[10] Controllable, acute medical emergencies allow health care practitioners to return the patient to a state of health such that the body does not limit the autonomy of the individual. In this way, the autonomous self is disembodied such that one's corporeal state is not understood as being integrated with one's sense of self. Indeed, as Bruce Jennings, Daniel Callahan, and Arthur Caplan (12) state, "The first component of the autonomy paradigm is a particular interpretation of the meaning of illness and the goal of medicine: illness is seen as an alien threat to the self, and the goal is to defend and restore the self by curing or compensating for the illness." The "true self," according to this autonomy paradigm, is the self un-encumbered by a disabled, chronically ill, or vulnerable body. The natural bodily state, then, is that of the normalized body, which does not interfere with the desires or ends of the self. On this view, one's autonomy, identity, and personal ends are prior to and independent of one's experience of ill-ness. It is as if illness were merely a physical state that interferes with the autonomy and self-identity of the ill person without being an *integral part* of that ill person's life; thus, if we can overcome illness through technology, we could preserve the unencumbered, autonomous self with which we all supposedly identify.[11]

What we fail to acknowledge with our paradigms of health, control, acute care, and autonomy is that these are not absolute states. Health varies in degree and can mark some areas of a person's life but not others. One can be healthy, for example, while experiencing the limitations imposed by a 90-year-old body; one can be physically healthy, yet live with paraplegia. Furthermore, patients may survive an acute medical emergency to remain chronically ill thereafter. Alternatively, a doctor can preserve lives in acute situations without providing cure. The bright lines drawn between health and illness or disability is recognized by some bioethicists as highly prob-lematic, since doctors may act to save a life but not provide a "cure" for the patient's ailments. In short, the medical world cannot be cleanly divided into acute versus chronic care or curative versus noncurative treatment (Moros et al.).

The acute care paradigm allows us to treat a patient's acute medical problem without the attendant mental and social components that consti-tute chronic care. A patient in an acute medical crisis is assumed to need only *medical* attention: The medical condition is definable, treatable, and controllable. Elderly people and others who require home care services, on the other hand, are not in a medically controllable condition, and their par-ticular problems usually have complex social and psychological facets. The acute care paradigm thus allows medicine to sidestep many sociomedical is-sues that arise within chronic care, such as loneliness, depression, poverty, lack of social support, nutrition concerns, the completion of mundane tasks, and the navigation of chronic pain and psychic suffering.

Here received notions of productivity come into play, since men are as-sociated with the typically "productive" work that is associated with the public sphere. In an ends-oriented culture that judges men's productivity by output—by the amount and quality of what they produce—engaging in caretaking is certain failure. Care work may not appear to be productive ac-tivity, especially when one is performing mundane tasks like bathing and feeding dependents, tasks that one must complete repeatedly. In this way, the acute care paradigm for health care lines up nicely with our broader masculinist cultural ideals, since the acute care model is also ends-oriented, focusing on the production of a normal, functioning body that is capable of returning to productive activity. The "nonproductive" work involved in chronic care—work which is, by our paradigm, futile, since no good is produced in the end—falls upon women, since they are still considered largely nonproductive.[12]

So, I am arguing, it is the constellation of factors like the role women have historically played in caretaking and the development of an acute care paradigm that have rendered the family so fundamental to the delivery of home care. These two factors are symbiotic, since chronic care needs are rendered shameful and private. Chronic care patients fail to meet the norms of autonomy, independence, and self-sufficiency that are still core to our liberal democratic society, thus resulting in the fulfillment of home care needs by women in their traditional private sphere of the home. As Holstein claims,

> In sum, policy and its omissions can explain why home care has become primarily a family responsibility. The gendered nature of the labor market offers some suggestion as to why "family" most often means women. Cultural values and assumptions, even ideologies, also support women's primary responsibility for caregiving. (235)

But home care's reliance on families to fulfill their loved ones' care needs has resulted not only in serious questions surrounding the gendered nature of caretaking but also in concerns about race and class.

### Race, Class, and Familial Care

So far I have argued that by appealing to "familial" caretaking, home care trades on a very traditional gendered division of labor. But this is not the end of the story: Embedded in the familial care expectation are issues of race and class. For example, while studies show that a quarter of American families are caring for an elderly relative at home, elderly blacks are twice as likely as whites to receive familial care. As I will indicate, the reasons for this are complex and involve both our history of racism in the United States as well as a strong familial ethic in the black community that emphasizes family and community connections. Ultimately, the issues of race and class that arise within the familial context only further problematize the current practice of home care in the United States. African American families carry a much greater burden of stress and economic hardship as well as lost wages, job opportunities, and educational opportunities.

While these hardships may be faced by *all* those caring for ill family members at home, the fact that blacks disproportionately meet these difficulties means that they face even greater setbacks associated with the caretaking burden.

Consider the example of Charles Mitchell, a police dispatcher at North Carolina Central University in Durham, who has chosen to work the graveyard shift so that he can be home during the day to take care of his aging mother. Mitchell has no paid home care aides or housekeepers to help care for his mother; but he has the help of family and friends. Mitchell's two sisters and girlfriend all take care of his mother. One sister stays with her while Mitchell works; the other sister regularly shows up to fix her mother's hair and provide intimate care. This caretaking arrangement—where family and other loved ones work together to care for the elderly—is typical of African American families.[13]

While some commentators, like James Blackwell, claim that racism and oppression bind African American communities together, there is a much stronger, positive reason for their strength of community. External oppression and suspicion of a medical system that has done violence to blacks are factors in the high rate of familial care by African American families, but such care is much more than just a reaction against oppression. It is an expression of a strong familial ethic that takes seriously respect for family and community. One adult daughter spent five years caring for her mother. When urged by her doctor to put her mother in a nursing home, she said, "We just don't do that. Not with our people."[14] As commentators note, "These values—among them, the primacy of family, the importance of education, and the necessity for individual enterprise and hard work—have been fundamental to black survival" (Franklin and Norton, 3–4). So despite theories that black families are fragmented and lack the "tie that binds," there is evidence of a very strong family structure within the black community.

But it is dangerous to overemphasize the familial ethic that undergirds the African American community. For in addition to this ethic, family members take on heavy burdens because they don't trust the medical system. And, indeed, this distrust is not misplaced, for medicine has a sorry history of using and abusing members of the black community. As Dorothy Roberts indicates, with the history of sickle-cell screening, the Tuskegee syphilis experiment, and involuntary sterilization, blacks "harbor a well-founded distrust" of both white physicians and our racist medical system (260). This distrust leads to the taking on of a heavy care responsibility by black families because of their refusal to place elderly family members in nursing homes and other long-term care institutions. And since many

African American families lack the resources to access the services of home health aides, they end up taking on the care burden alone. Add to this a lack of education and access to education (in some cases), and one further sees how much more difficult it becomes for blacks to obtain Medicaid and Medicare benefits. Many don't know when they are entitled to health care services and how to collect it.

Clearly, then, home health care raises issues of class as well as race, since the middle class is far more likely to have the resources to pay for home care services for elderly family members. In addition, middle-class whites do not share the same suspicion of the medical profession as blacks, making them much more comfortable in utilizing services like nursing homes and in following the advice of doctors. For example, in the past, discrimination and poverty prevented blacks from entering nursing homes in North Carolina. Homes that they could afford, when they were allowed entry, offered poor care at best.[15] These inequalities must be factored in when considering the ethics of familial home care, since caretaking becomes not just a familial burden of care but a racialized one as well.

Furthermore, when considering home health care, a traditional conception of "family" should not be invoked. If we want to be maximally inclusive in our ethical treatment of home care, we should not appeal to the paradigm of the married, middle- to upper-class woman in a heterosexual relationship. While privileged middle-class women linked to economically powerful men may also be familial caretakers, this should not be taken as the norm. On the contrary, the circumstances of some American men prevent them from playing a large economic role in the support of their families. As Twila Perry indicates, disparities between white and black students attending college, statistics on the number of black men in prison, and unemployment statistics for black men indicate how difficult it is for them to play a dominant economic role in their families. Indeed, many African American families are now headed by single women, so the effects of institutionalized racism make the middle-class nuclear family an unlikely arrangement for many American families. Indeed, blacks are much less likely than whites to have spouses who can help with their care.

As a result, grandmothers in black communities are increasingly doing care work for their grandchildren. Thus, the familial ethic to which I referred grounds not only the care of elderly family members by younger ones but also the care of young family members by elderly ones. So when considering caretaking within black families, the care work done by elderly members must not be overlooked; for our purposes, this means that the elderly individuals in need of home care services are themselves caretakers, and their care work, too, is worthy of recognition and remuneration. By understanding family in the traditional ideological way, then, we also rely on social inequalities and outdated demographics that provide the wrong picture of both the family and family caretaking.

Martha Fineman's approach to paid family caretaking rejects such a privileged conception of the family. Her policy recommendation rejects the centrality of men to social structures of caretaking, and dismisses the notion that caretaking is accomplished within a privatized family structure. Rather, she sees caretaking as a public concern and refuses to look to men for caretaker support. Fineman requires the state, not individual men within the privacy of their families, to provide financial support for caretakers. Her account of women's care work, then, is responsive to black women, single women, and lesbians who do not fit the paradigm of the traditional nuclear family. For example, white middle-class women are unfairly advantaged by their ability to do care work at home, with full spousal support. Perry writes approvingly of Fineman's approach:

> A theory in which the perceived rights of women are not dependent on their relationships to men places the choices of women not attached to men or attached to low-income men on the same level as choices of women who are linked to men who have money. (156)

The high rate of at-home care by black family members may be a labor of love—and may be wrapped up within an ethic of family and community—but it has serious results for individuals with few resources to begin with. Black caretakers tend to have less money than white families caring for an elderly family member, so they bear a disproportionate burden of care. Since they cannot afford to hire paid caretakers, they do the work themselves. In addition, more than half of all black caretakers have children under 18 at home who also require care; this compares with 39 percent of all white caretakers. And statistics show that, of the over-65 age group, 34 percent of blacks live in a multigenerational home, compared with only 18 percent of whites.[16]

No account of the ethics of home care is complete, then, if it fails to address issues of race and class. Later in this book I will consider fully the notion of women's care work as a subsidy to the state and its capacity to address these issues of race and class. Such a notion rejects the typical view of the middle-class, heterosexual, two-parent family, and instead allows for any number of family caretaking arrangements. I will contend that the model of caretaking as recognized and remunerable is best, not only because it is inclusive of black family formations but also because it includes single-parent and nonheterosexual family formations.

Issues of race and class do not only arise within the area of family care-taking. They are also central to any consideration of paid, formal home care services.

### The Provision of Formal Care

For the remainder of this chapter I will treat the ethical issues in paid caretaking. In considering the provision of paid, formal home care, I will focus specifically on home health aides. While there are other key players involved (including nurses, physiotherapists, and occupational therapists), we need to consider the situation of the worst-off workers in the home care industry. To give an accurate and inclusive account of the ethics of home care, we must start with the lowest paid, "lowliest" workers to understand what is wrong with the system and why it is largely unethical.

With the advent of DRGs increasing the demand for services, the home care industry has been plagued with problems surrounding the hiring and retention of home care workers.[17] Given the poor working conditions associated with the home health aide's job, including low wages, physical and emotional stress, lack of benefits, and uncertainty of hours, home care providers have had a hard time recruiting workers. Those who are recruited are generally poor minority women who lack the educational or skilled training to obtain more secure and lucrative forms of employment. And in a market where the bottom line involves cutting costs and increasing profits, home care providers have incentives to exploit their workforce by keeping wages extremely low, refusing to provide benefits (including health care insurance, vacation pay, or sick leave), and failing to provide stable, constant hours for their home care workers. In addition, home care providers rely heavily on families of their clients to provide the "supplemental" care that is necessary to maintain the client in her home.

To get an idea of the problems that plague home care aides, consider an example. Mary is a 30-year-old woman from the West Indies who has been working as a home care aide for the past two years. Before beginning as an aide, Mary took a one-week preparatory course that provided her with all the basic skills necessary for caring for individuals in their homes. She was trained in how to transfer clients from bed to wheelchair, in changing bedding while the patient was in bed, in giving bed baths, in turning bedridden patients to prevent bedsores, and in providing adequate nutritional meals for clients with diminished appetites. She has received no special training to work with clients who are suffering from terminal cancer or AIDS or who have paraplegia or quadriplegia.

At first, Mary was only offered shifts that fell within the scope of her training. She worked with clients who required light housekeeping, bathing, dressing, and meals. But over time she is finding that the care coordinators at the office are asking her to care for clients who are well beyond her skill level. Two months ago, she was sent to the home of a man with quadriplegia, where she was expected to work an hydraulic lift, change and sanitize urine bags, and treat mild bedsores (all for which she has no training). A week ago she was sent to the home of a woman who is dying of stomach cancer. The client needed help administering her morphine, which Mary was not legally entitled to do.

Mary thinks all this is bad enough, but in addition she is not being paid the extra money that is supposed to go with these increased responsibilities. She is also not paid for her travel time to and from these clients' homes. Sometimes her scheduled shifts are so short—two or three hours—that it costs her more in babysitting fees than she earns in doing the shift. And she worries about getting sick, since that means she will be off work without pay and she has no medical insurance. Mary is paid only $5.56 per hour.

As this example shows, caretakers remain so poorly paid that one can see them as little more than paid volunteers. A large proportion of home care workers in the United States are minority women, including new immigrants from the Caribbean Islands. Many home care workers and their families are economically deprived. One study indicates that 80 percent of workers reported they were unable to afford adequate housing, and 35 percent indicate that they are sometimes unable to buy enough food for their families.[18]

Indeed, that home care is dominated by minority women is in part what renders it a new "job ghetto," since where an immigrant workforce is available, wages are notoriously low and the jobs are unusually demanding.[19] That a large number of those in the home care workforce are poorly educated women who sometimes do not speak English means that the work is considered "unskilled" and is therefore poorly remunerated.

Traditional economic theory suggests that long-term labor shortages in competitive markets will not persist, given the mechanism of supply and demand. When employers cannot find workers through whom to offer their services, they increase wages to stimulate the market and so attract more laborers. Such increases raise the price of service to consumers, who then lower their service demands. This combination of supply and demand results in a balanced labor market, as the increased worker supply and lowered demand restore stability to the market (Feldman, 163).

But traditional economic theory cannot address the problems in home health care because the home care market is an imperfect one. Competitive behavior is thwarted by Medicare and Medicaid payment regulations, and the care work is devalued by the refusal to see it as work. This is why the home care industry has not responded to the workforce paucity by simply offering more money to workers.

The home care industry cannot lure workers into jobs through economic incentives. This is in part because providers must keep wages down because of DRG limits and low Medicare/Medicaid reimbursements. The more home care aides are paid, the more quickly the finite funds offered by Medicare or Medicaid are eaten up. Indeed, despite the demand for aides, a rise in wages is not forthcoming: Rather than consumers paying for the services and paying the market price for them, it is usually government agencies that are footing the bill. Since caps are placed on Medicare and Medicaid reimbursements, this means that the system of supply and demand simply does not work. If home care agencies offer aides anything like a decent, living wage, they will quickly go bankrupt.

These market considerations have had a grave impact on the stability of the home care workforce. As studies indicate, agencies are reporting extremely high employee turnover rates as well as worker shortages in some parts of the country. Indeed, some authors put the average turnover rate at 60–70 percent.[20] The result of this movement through the home care system is that client care is detrimentally impacted, so both caretakers and clients are the victims of this chaotic system of care.

Home care aides move in and out of different agencies and the home care industry, just as physicians shift from one health maintenance organization to another. In both health care and home health care, the system of managed care has led to a constant shift of doctors and aides in and out of different agencies. Thus, the home care industry is unstable in large part because it currently functions within the managed care ethos. Like doctors, aides are discouraged from forming relationships with clients due to the revolving door of providers and patients who move in and out of the system. The problems with home health care, then, are easily viewed as an extension of the problem of managed care, for just as managed care practice results in high turnover rates between doctor-patient-HMO, so it results in high turnover rates between home care agency-client-aide.

The problems with home care are systemic and should be viewed as such. While the industry does suffer from problems of poor caretaking, high turnover rates, and client abuse, these problems are connected to the market-driven managed care system of health care provision within which home care is practiced. As I will argue in chapter 6, to make home care ethical, we need to take a hard look at the way that health care in general is provided in the United States.

But first, let us consider the philosophies that undergird the practice of home health care. As I will argue in the following chapter, differing philosophies of home care, though largely unrecognized, are expressed via current practice and by home care's placement within a system of managed care. Furthermore, the philosophies expressed by agencies and caretakers/clients are in conflict, as personal relationships clash with the demands of the market.

# 2 Examining Philosophies of Home Care

The preceding chapter detailed home health care as it is currently practiced. As I indicated, home care is premised on the notion that it is a cheaper alternative to institution-based care, that people prefer to be cared for in their homes rather than in institutions, and that home care services must follow the example of the broader U.S. managed care system.

This chapter will address philosophies of home care. That there *are* philosophies undergirding home care has not received much notice, yet there are central values expressed in the way home care is overseen and carried out.[1] But these values are not consistent, because they are not expressed on only one level. On the contrary, there are different parties, from the organizational level down to field workers, acting out different values in home care. For example, central values—that go to the core of what home care stands for, the purpose it is meant to serve, and the individuals to whom it applies—are rooted in the corporate, market-driven managed care model of care provision. Yet there are different values embedded in the *practice* of home care, where caretakers and clients express a noncommodified, non-contractual understanding of their relationships. Any discourse surrounding the philosophy of home care, then, is complicated by conflicting value systems and ideologies of home care that mask values upheld in practice. We need to sort out the philosophies that exist on different levels to be clear about what home care values are and to determine in praxis what they should be.

On one level, the central values of home care—that is, the corporate values on which the practice of home care is based—fail to address the real needs of clients and to understand the phenomenology of illness and dependency. Home care's corporate values focus on washing and dressing bodies, feeding mouths, preventing bedsores, and transferring bodies from bed to wheelchair and back again. While such activities can be performed in a more or less caring manner, the actual corporate values of home care do not require that those who care for clients should care *about* them as well.[2] I will explore this critique and suggest that the ideal values surrounding home care can and should be different. What home care accomplishes is not just washing and feeding bodies (though this is certainly a part of its practice). Rather, as Arthur Frank has pointed out, the experience of illness and incapacity requires a human response to the individual's care needs. And having clean bodies is only a small part of what home care recipients need.

To understand philosophies of home care, I will consider the following questions: What are the central values of home care? Who determines them? How can we identify them? I will also herein consider questions such as: Who is served by the practice of home care? What good do we do in providing it? and What are the decision-making relationships involved? But first let us understand what "central values" are.

## Central Values Testing in Home Care

David Ozar and David Sokol have pursued the issue of central values testing in their work on dental ethics. They indicate that any profession expresses central values through its practices and that "no professional group is expected by the larger community to be expert in their clients' *entire* well-being" (56). Indeed, to expect a profession (medical doctors, for example) to secure in toto the values of its clients would be expecting too much and would place undue strain on practitioners. Still, as Ozar and Sokol point out,

> There is always necessarily a certain limited set of values that are the specific focus of each profession's expertise, and it is therefore the principal job and obligation of that profession to secure these for its clients. These values can be called the *central values* of that profession's practice. (56)

Determining the central values of home health care is a complex endeavor, since home care lacks any clearly defined norms and there is a gap between its purported values and those that are exhibited in practice. Furthermore, it is not clear who counts as practitioners and as "professionals" in the field. While it may seem obvious that home health aides are the practitioners in question, I will indicate in what follows that these field workers have little impact on forming and informing the central values of home health care. This is because home health care is practiced without an ongoing dialogue that involves field workers; hence the gap I mentioned between the corporate values of home care and those that are evidenced in practice. Yet despite these difficulties, it is important to determine how a corporate philosophy supports the practice of home health care, in order to understand why it has manifest itself in its particular form.

Ozar and Sokol indicate that, to do central values testing, one must start with the conduct and discourse of the members of the profession as they pertain to practice. In the case of the dental profession, this means examining the conduct of dentists and their patients "as these parties discuss and then make decisions about dental treatment" (57). Beyond this, one would also examine codes of ethics as the stated mission and values of a practice. For example, in the medical and nursing professions one finds codes of ethics that proscribe certain activities (lying to patients and violating patient autonomy) and that mandate others (in the case of nurses, acting as patient advocate). By focusing on conduct and discourse, we can understand how values are both enacted and talked about within the profession in question.

In a similar vein, Margaret Walker's *Moral Understandings: A Feminist Study in Ethics* lays the foundations for the kind of investigation of home care's central values that I have in mind. Walker argues that morality is a collaborative effort taken up by communities that share what she calls "moral understandings." She describes these understandings in the following way:

> In all of its expressions, morality is fundamentally *interpersonal;* it arises out of and is reproduced or modified in what goes on between or among people. In this way, morality is collaborative; we construct and sustain it together. . . . What goes on morally between people is constrained and made intelligible by a background of understandings about what people are supposed to do, expect, and understand. These are the "moral understandings" of my title. Self-direction, responsiveness to others, and mutual accountability are constant tasks in human social life, but the ways that human societies shape these vary. Particular understandings are revealed in the daily rounds of interaction that show how people make sense of their own and others' responsibilities in terms of their identities, relationships, and values. But we have to *look* in order to see them. (10)

That the moral understandings of a community are shared, but not always obvious, is important in this context. For this means that we may engage in practices with little clarity about the beliefs, values, and assumptions that back them up. And, as I will argue, this is certainly true in the home care context: At the very time that home care is carried out, we are engaging shared understandings of which we may not be explicitly aware. By stepping back to examine these understandings, we can determine their worth in practice and consider other, more fitting ones.

Thus, Ozar, Sokol, and Walker's approaches are similar in that they consider how values are expressed by discourse and practice. The former focus on central values expressed within professions, while Walker considers more broadly the way that certain values are expressed by their practice within a community. In considering the central values expressed by home health care, I will adopt these authors' strategies. Through this investigation, then, I will address the philosophies of home care.

### Professional Roles in Home Health Care

To understand its central values, let us begin with the professional roles in home health care. Consider Ozar and Sokol's claim that "no professional group is expected by the larger community to be expert in their clients' *entire* well-being." This claim is problematized within the home care arena, where workers are, indeed, expected to be expert in their clients' entire well-being. Home care services run such a wide gamut that they cover all aspects of clients' lives: physical, emotional, nutritional, social, and economic.[3] Indeed, Lenard Kaye understands professionalism in home care as including a wide range of roles and activities. She points out that good practice includes affective or psychologically supportive roles and instrumental functions. Furthermore, as she notes, home care crosses disciplinary lines, so that even professionals like occupational therapists and social workers provide psychological and physical care. But the roles and responsibilities played by the home care practitioner still relate back to their disciplinary backgrounds. So, for example, if the practitioner is a home health care nurse, her likely emphasis will be on performance of physical tasks such as changing dressings, colostomy care, catheter insertion, and monitoring vital signs. Alternatively, if the practitioner is a social worker, she is likely to assume responsibility for providing program coordination and supervision, counseling and client advocacy, and overseeing administrative responsibilities.

Kaye's account assumes that home care workers hold professional status and that we can recognize the roles and responsibilities that attach to such professional status. And indeed, if we focus on the professions of nursing and social work, we can identify these elements as they relate to good nursing or social work practice in home health care. But the notion of a "professional" role that has been highlighted by Ozar and Sokol and echoed by Kaye overlooks a key role in home health care that is marked by non-professional status: the home care aide. Such home care workers, as I indicated in chapter 1, lack professional status. Their job is poorly defined, and the work is considered unskilled and sustaining. In his 1998 essay, Michael Bayles has distinguished professional from nonprofessional work by pointing to three necessary features of professional activity: extensive training, training that involves a considerable intellectual element, and training that provides an important community service. Recognized professions also share features such as processes of certification, organizations of members (for example, the American Medical Association), and professional autonomy. Home care aides, as they are commonly understood, exhibit none of these features. Rather, they perform duties that are functionally diverse and that are sustaining rather than interventive. So where a physician intervenes in a medical emergency and then steps back, home care aides do the repetitive, sustaining work to maintain a client in her daily life.[4] More significantly, home care aides are not identified with a body of knowledge that must be "mastered" in order to do the job well. On the contrary, the knowledge exhibited by home care aides is considered to be "common knowledge" and so of no particular value in terms of service to community.

As I am arguing, home care lacks its *own* understanding of the home care worker's role, since the kinds of professional roles addressed by Kaye attach to other professions and are only derivatively associated with home care. So, for example, while a home care nurse will no doubt adhere to the role and responsibilities associated with her profession, they come from her profession and not from home health care itself. The same is certainly true for any other home care practitioner affiliated with a profession: She will understand her role in connection with her profession and not with home care itself.

That there is no professional role associated solely with home health aides means that such workers suffer invisibility and lack a voice in formulating formal rules and responsibilities surrounding the practice of home health care. But if we look more closely at their conduct and discourse, we see that aides express in their daily practice a role identification and an understanding of responsibility that comes out of home care practice *itself*.

For example, aides usually act to protect the client, not the home care provider. This is because they know, from working with real individuals with real lives, that home care is not about washing bodies or feeding mouths; it is about caring for a whole person with a past, present, and future. By virtue of their work in the private sphere of the home, aides come to understand clients in their real, lived, social context. And where those actual persons come up against an impersonal system that metes out care based on economic considerations rather than clients' needs, aides may find themselves lying for clients (for example, noting improvements in the client's functioning) in order to ensure they continue to receive care and to continue the valued relationship.[5] Within the context of managed care, where the focus is on cost-cutting, such responses by home care aides are simply human responses to human needs. And this response, I want to argue, is an expression of the health care aide's role and responsibilities. Yet this conduct contravenes the most obvious value exhibited by the home care industry: profitability.

### Profits and Home Care

Profitability is another major value expressed by the home care industry. The move to home care would never have taken place had it not initially been seen as an economically viable (indeed, profitable) option. To the extent that home care is paid for by Medicare or Medicaid, it has attracted for-profit companies with an interest in making money. These companies have displaced small, community-based home care services that focus on service to clients, putting them out of business because they cannot compete with the large corporations that contain divisions of home health services.

Critics could respond that home care has not proven as profitable as had initially been hoped. Indeed, home health care providers are currently at risk of providing services to clients without remuneration because of limits placed by Medicare/Medicaid on reimbursable services. But this does not answer the question of what values are found in home health care, for whether or not it is currently proving profitable, profitability is one of the key values that home care upholds.

The way in which home care services are allocated expresses the value of profitability. Consider, for example, needs assessments, which are tools used to indicate the needs of particular clients in setting up their home care services. These assessments, using tools like OARS (Older Americans Research and Services), the CARE methodology, or MAI (Multilevel Assessment Inventory), incorporate measures of physical health, ADLs (activities of daily living), mental health, social resources, and economic status. By assessing potential clients on these grounds, home care providers develop a care plan for the home care client.

The result of such assessments, however, is not the provision of care that clients need, but provision of services that are deemed affordable by the providers. Note that providers are themselves limited by Medicaid and Medicare reimbursements: Even if a client is assessed as needing full-time or near full-time care, she simply will not receive it. As Robert Hudson points out, the purpose of home care services is not to meet the needs of clients but to reduce reliance on hospitals for patient care. As he states,

> The purpose of Medicare's home health benefit was focused . . . on the desire to reduce hospital stays. Thus, for Medicare purposes, home health services were defined as skilled, intermittent, part-time services provided under a physician's written direction and plan of care in the residence of the homebound client. (277–78)

Thus, the purpose of needs assessments is undermined by the strict limits placed on reimbursable home care services. And since most Americans cannot afford to pay out-of-pocket for their home care needs, they must accept the care hours allotted. In addition, clients' families fill in the gaps between the needs assessment and the care that is actually provided. What becomes clear through such a process is the value of cost savings and profitability to home health care.

It is unsurprising, then, under the current circumstances of home care practice that clients, families, and home care aides may see themselves as bound together against an impersonal and exploitative system.

## The Value of Caring for Bodies

Another value expressed by the home care industry is that of caring for bodies that require washing, dressing, feeding, and toileting. It is important, again, to distinguish between the values expressed by home care aides and those indicated by the industry itself, for it is my contention that there is a difference between the values stated by the industry and those practiced by workers in the field. For instance, as Joan Tronto indicates, there is a difference between caring *for* a client, that is, seeing to her physical needs, and caring *about* her, or providing attentive, loving care that is responsive to her articulated needs. Caring about someone may also involve perceiving another's needs without distorting them via one's own perceptions. In this, says Tronto, one finds the moral quality of care (1998, 16). Thus, the value expressed by the home care industry is in caring for clients' bodies and not in caring about them in the moral sense Tronto has in mind. While caring for bodies certainly must be accomplished in the home care field, this is surely not all that is required for a rich philosophy of home care.

One need only encounter a narrative like that of Arthur Frank to understand why the value of caring for bodies is inadequate to the practice of home health care. Frank experienced life-threatening illnesses that unexpectedly dropped him into the world of medicine; his account of his treatment within the medical system indicates the system's inability to care about patients. As Frank articulates it,

> I reserve the name "caregivers" for the people who are willing to listen to ill persons and to respond to their individual experiences. Caring has nothing to do with categories; it shows the person that her life is valued because it recognizes what makes her experience particular. One person has no right to categorize another, but we do have the privilege of coming to understand how each of us is unique. When the caregiver communicates to the ill person that she cares about that uniqueness, she makes the person's life meaningful. And as that person's life story becomes part of her own, the caregiver's life is made meaningful as well. Care is inseparable from understanding, and like understanding, it must be symmetrical. Listening to another, we hear ourselves. Caring for another, we either care for ourselves as well, or we end in burnout and frustration. (48)

Frank addresses the importance of caring about people in home care from both the perspective of the care recipient and the caretaker. The value of care isn't expressed only in one's physical ministrations to others but also in the give-and-take of a mutual relationship. As he points out, caring for others involves care for self; without this reciprocal relationship, caretakers become frustrated and they burn out.

In a similar vein, Seyla Benhabib has distinguished between what she calls the "generalized" and the "concrete" other. Like Frank, Benhabib argues that in both theory and practice we have focused on the "generalized other," that is, viewing other persons as rational beings entitled to the same rights and duties that we hold. By taking this standpoint, argues Benhabib, we abstract from the concrete realities of the individual's life and fail to recognize her individuality. On the generalized model, human relationships are reduced to concerns for *formal equality* and *reciprocity*, without concern for the individual vagaries of human life. Taking the standpoint of the concrete other, however, requires the kind of attentiveness to the individual as a particular person that Frank is concerned about. While we do, indeed, view each concrete individual as a rational being worthy of respect, we also see her with a unique history, identity, and psycho-social constitution (Benhabib 1987, 164). In so doing, we engage in a kind of reciprocity, but not a reciprocity of the generalized, formal sort. Rather, it is the kind of reciprocity that Frank is getting at in the passage cited above.[6] As both Benhabib and Frank highlight, one cannot sustain for long the contentless relationship between self and "generalized other"; rather, we need to understand others in their uniqueness, listen to ill persons, and, as Frank puts it, "respond to their individual experiences." In so doing, both care recipient and caretaker's lives are made meaningful.

Thus, the high rate of caretaker "burn out" in home care that I outlined in chapter 1 is telling. It suggests two things: first, that home care aides are not given the luxury of time to care about clients in the moral sense that Tronto and Frank address; and second, that the kind of symmetrical reciprocity highlighted by Benhabib that is part of good, concrete care relationships is lacking in home care situations. Since corporate values are not supportive of this kind of care relationship, aides are denied the fulfilling experience of reciprocal care, lack the self-care that goes with it, and end up exhausted (both physically and emotionally), desperate, and angry. Aides cannot sustain this situation for long, and so they move from agency to agency, in and out of the home care industry, at alarming rates.

Importantly, then, the corporate values that home care officially upholds fail to address the "meaning-making" that is part of home care practice. Those engaged in the give-and-take of care are engaged in creating meaning—purpose—in one another's lives. By focusing on caring for bodies, corporate values reduce home care to its bare mechanics, robbing both clients and caretakers of the most meaningful, and fulfilling, aspect of the relationship. To do this, I am arguing, is to morally wrong those engaged in home care practice.

### An Acute Care Model

Connie Zuckerman, Nancy Dubler, and Bart Collopy point out that home care is a form of chronic care, since it seeks to make people as independent as possible without reversing their medical conditions or providing cure (13). Yet while these authors are right that home care *is* chronic care, it nevertheless expresses the value of acute medical interventions. Chapter 1 detailed the relationship between home care and acute care interventions: I argued that, just like the broader arena of health care, it values an acute care model of care provision. Home care is viewed from the perspective of acute care interventions rather than the more fitting chronic care model for two main reasons: first, because an acute care model better allows for limitations placed on care, and second, because such an approach upholds the important cultural values of autonomy, independence, and self-sufficiency. With regard to the first point, consider the costs involved with meeting clients' chronic care needs: Care would be indefinite, multifaceted, and intensive, requiring attention to their economic situations, their physical surroundings, mental state, and their permanent physical ailments. There is no cure, for example, for aging, which factors into the need for home care services. By adhering to an acute care model, then, home care sidesteps these demands, limiting care to clients who have been discharged from hospitals, and who are ill enough to be home-bound. Because interventions are short-term and limited in scope, clients' socioeconomic situations need not be taken into account in the plan of care.

With regard to the latter point, an acute care paradigm serves the broader society within which home care is practiced, since it allows us to uphold the myth of autonomy and self-control that is core to the American ethos. If home care were to embrace a chronic care paradigm, it would be admitting to the frailty of the human condition; to the inevitability of aging, disability, dependency, and chronic illness. Given the way in which contemporary medicine resists association with these realities, and given home health care's patterning on the broader system of managed care, it is not surprising that home care evidences these same values. Again, it is at the organizational level that the emphasis on acute care interventions is expressed, given the kinds of restrictions and limitations set on home care services. Field workers know all too well the actual, sometimes mundane, chronic care needs of home care clients.

### The Value of Loyalty

The home care industry expresses the value of worker loyalty to the provider rather than to the actual clients served. This value is evidenced by both policy and practice, and it was part of my own experience. Many of the protocols set out in my home care training were premised on my commitment to the organization and its rules. The charting requirement, for example, served the home care agency by having the aides chart where (and whether) improvements were evident in the clients' eating patterns, mobility, strength, and mental state. Indications that clients were not improving or that their abilities were worsening served as grounds for the agency to terminate care of the client. Furthermore, the agency for which I worked prohibited certain activities in clients' homes: for example, I could not change lightbulbs if it required my standing on a chair or ladder, I could damp mop but not hand wash floors, and I could steady a client's hand to help get her medications in her mouth, but I was not allowed to place the pills in her mouth myself. While there may be legitimate reasons for such rules, they were premised on the understanding that my loyalties were with the agency, not with the client. I did not feel such loyalty to my home care agency, however: Rather, I more often identified with the clients themselves.

I would not leave an elderly female client alone in her home with a dark hallway, even if it required my standing on a chair to change the lightbulb; I would hand wash floors for clients when they did not have a mop available (indeed, many were too poor to have proper cleaning supplies like mops, buckets, and cleansers); and since it meant the difference between staying at home or being put in a nursing facility, I would put their medications in their mouths when they were unable to do so themselves.[7] In my view, these accommodations were basic to caring about, and not just caring for, clients. In an almost endless variety of home settings, with different personalities and needs involved, rule-bound care delivery can be highly obstructive.[8]

Thus, while loyalty should, indeed, be a central value in home care, the question remains: loyal to whom? Based on a corporate model of home care, field workers owe their loyalties to the agencies that employ them; indeed, worker loyalty is cultivated by most businesses. But in the arena of home health care, loyalties may shift to the clients, who are often vulnerable, caught in and abandoned by an impersonal system that uses them to cut costs and generate revenue.

### The Value of Familial Love

Home care places a premium on family caretaking: Without such free care provision, the home care system would fall apart. In the economic sense, at least, families are valued and central to a corporate philosophy of home care.

But if we scratch below the surface we see that families are not valued in a manner that encourages a rich philosophy of home care: That is, they are instrumentally valued, but not treated as having intrinsic worth. The state trades on notions of altruistic care, intimacy, familial bonds, and filial love—all aspects of families that we generally consider to be inherently valuable—in order to call forth a supply of female caretakers in service to the state. And though familial care is not usually understood in this way, in chapter 3 I will argue that it *should* be. When female kin provide care to their family members, they are engaging in service to the state; since it is a hidden subsidy, we fail to see it as such. Of course, understanding familial caretaking in this way does not preclude the kinds of loving, altruistic relationships we generally associate with families. On the contrary, it protects such relationships by ensuring that families are not destroyed by an extreme burden of care.

As James and Hilde Lindemann Nelson argue, the "instrumental use of love is incoherent. Love's fundamental presupposition is that the beloved is

to be cherished, not used" (45). The home care industry's appeal to familial love is most offensive, then, on the grounds that the value is called in
service to instrumental purposes, often resulting in the rending of that love.
Families can be deeply harmed by care demands that have a damaging economic, social, and psychological impact. If the state truly cherished the familial role, family members would not be used and abused to the point
where the family is torn apart.

Familial love is, however, a central value in home care and should be
seen as such. While the state and the home care industry give lip service to
the importance of familial love, field workers and family members know its
deeper value. Clients do not use their family's love as a means to receiving
free care; while loving relationships may result in physical caretaking as an
expression of care, it should not be extorted from families. *To treat seriously familial love as a central value in home care we must provide support
networks that allow and encourage families to engage in caretaking or that
free them from caretaking in order to do other activities that serve their
loved ones, such as paid employment.*

Aide/client relationships are similarly rewarding because a kind of familial love often develops as the relationship endures. As Tracy Karner
phrases it, home care workers become "fictive kin" given the home setting,
the intimate details of the clients' lives to which workers become privy, and
the extremely personal tasks in which workers are engaged. In Karner's
study, home care supervisors warned workers against getting too close to
clients; as she claims,

> The administrative staff is concerned with the negative repercussions that
> can come from the ambiguities of social exchanges. The friendship and
> caring between worker and client can imply additional obligations and du-
> ties, as the expectations of friends for assistance are higher than those for
> a paid worker. However, despite the discouragement of staff, the home
> care workers continue to become attached to their clients. As this deepens,
> the bond that comes from a sharing of selves facilitates the adoption stage
> where both parties "adopt" the other as a family member. (76)

Again, from the organizational level we can see the dis-value of these kinds
of bonds: As businesses, home care agencies have a vested interest in workers and clients not forming them. Solidarity with the agency is crucial for
several reasons: first, to ensure that workers follow the formalized rules;
second, to keep workers on board with the mission to limit hours and wean
clients off care; third, to prevent the burnout that comes with workers getting too involved in clients' lives;[9] and fourth, to protect the agency against
legal problems that could stem from such a bond (for example, when el-

derly clients give gifts to workers, and family members accuse the worker of "stealing" from the elderly client). In short, "fictive kin" relationships get messy and complicated, and rather than being valued by home care employers, they are seen as undesirable complications.

The central corporate values of home care focus on profitability, acute care, loyalty, and the exploitation of familial love. These values are all understood instrumentally at the organizational level; how they translate into care for home care clients is a separate question that I will pursue in what follows. By adopting an acute care model, home care fails to see clients as whole persons with particular pasts, presents, and futures. The work of home care aides is also reduced to washing and dressing bodies, feeding mouths, and changing dressings. Clients become objects to be cared for rather than subjects to be cared about.

### The Mechanics of Home Care Delivery

A good example of the way in which home care is organized around a "mechanical" model of care is the small time allotments given to aides to help clients out of bed, bathe, perform toiletries, dress, and eat breakfast. In some cases, my morning shifts to aid clients with such ADLs and IADLs were only one hour long. Unsurprisingly, I found it impossible to accomplish these tasks in one hour, especially on days when my clients were not inclined to get out of bed or in cases where they could only move slowly. In order to even come close to the one-hour limit, I had to put clients through the mechanics of these tasks without much exchanging of pleasantries. I understood my task to be one of getting clients set for the day: Our morning rituals could set the tone for their entire day, and rushing clients through their toiletries hardly seemed like a good way to start off. Yet the home care office treated my job as the mechanical one of getting a body out of bed, washed, and dressed. How else could they justify a one-hour time limit to accomplish these tasks? I never could keep within my one-hour limit, as I found it impossible and distasteful to reduce my job—and my clients—to the mechanics of caring for a body. As Robin Fiore points out,

> While home care may give the appearance of enhancing personal control because the care recipient is not physically residing in an institution, home care is thick with institutional structure and controls. All aspects of care are strictly under the control of a third party; the services available are, of necessity, quite restrictive and the delivery of care is regimented rather than individualized. (254)

Fiore is right that organizational values regiment home care delivery; however, in most cases, aides do not express this value in their actual practice. On the contrary, as Karner notes in her study of home care workers, tasks are performed in the "context of a human dyad" (75).

The central values in home health care are in conflict, dictated from the top down by an impersonal and multilayered set of agencies (Medicare, Medicaid, health maintenance organizations, and home care agencies) to a disempowered workforce. The sometimes "warm and fuzzy" values to which the industry appeals—familial love, loyalty—are invoked for instrumental purposes like cost savings. But often the way in which field workers carry out their work indicates an "underground" system of values that displace corporate ones, what philosopher-historian Michel Foucault would call a counterdiscourse.

The account of home care I have given thus far can be fleshed out by appeal to the work of Foucault, who has offered scathing critiques of our major social institutions. Foucault's work forces us to question the obviousness and naturalness of our social structures, our ways of talking, and our social institutions (like medicine, schools, prisons, and "mad houses"). He urges us to accept the way in which seemingly natural facts (in this case, caretaking) are social constructions, or interpretations. But most importantly, perhaps, Foucault leads us to consider the ways in which subjects are managed, not just through restrictions and prohibitions, but, as Carlos Prado puts it,

> through enabling conceptions, definitions, and descriptions that generate and support behavior-governing norms. What is also new, and intellectually jarring, is [his] description of this degree of management as requiring the complicity of those managed. Complicity is required because what needs to be achieved . . . is the deep internalization of a carefully orchestrated value-laden understanding of the self. (55)

What this means for the institution of home care is that not only home care agencies but workers and clients *themselves* participate in the construction and maintenance of behavior-governing norms that are foundational to home care practice. That is, in the daily carrying-out of their work, aides are complicit in the very norms that serve to marginalize and oppress them. And perhaps this relates to the crazy-making and burnout that is part of aide work, for, as I have argued, aides resist and reject and at the same time live out and reinforce the norms surrounding home health care. How can this be?

First of all, according to Foucault, power is never totalizing or complete. This means it presupposes that those over whom power is exercised can resist; it exists only where there is potential resistance. Power only exists in its active application against resistance, and because to have power over someone means they are allowed some initiative, it can then become resistance. Prado says, "Power constrains *actions,* not individuals. Power is a totality made up of individuals being dominated, coerced, or intimidated; of individuals submitting to domination, coercion, or intimidation; and of individuals resisting domination, coercion, or intimidation" (37). Thus, the idea is not that aides and clients are simply dominated by the power of home care institutions; they can also resist.

Power is not merely something that functions negatively to oppress individuals; it is essential to the positive empowerment of resisting agents as well. Agents take advantage of existing techniques, strategies, and discourses to take initiative in reinvesting them with a power and meaning that is more affirming of their own sense of who they would like to be. Judith Butler has taken up this issue of power and indicated the multifarious ways in which we can parade or lampoon existing power structures in order to expose and "denaturalize" them.

So home care aides exhibit both complicity with and resistance to the corporate home care system. As I have argued, they resist the power structures through the forming of kinlike bonds with their clients, and by refusing to adhere to the rules for practice that come from the top down. Conversely, aides are also complicit with the system in a variety of ways. For example, they may participate in the competitive home care system by acting *as* competitors, working against one another to gain favor with clients and supervisors. It is common for aides to complain about one another to clients ("I wish Susan would finish the laundry during her shift instead of leaving it for me") or to supervisors ("Susan isn't finishing up her work during her shifts"). Aides sometimes accept the corporate conception of home care by allowing themselves to be divided and cut off from one another, thus only strengthening the sense that they are working in competition against one another. In this way, they both reject and reinforce the corporate norms governing home care, and they resist and internalize the power relations at work. Yet this is not as inconsistent as it sounds. As Foucault claims, power exists where there is potential resistance, and the site of home care is, indeed, a site of potential resistance.

But this is not where a Foucauldian analysis of home care ends. Issues of power and resistance enter into other areas of home care. For instance, the abuse by some aides of their clients, when understood from this Foucauldian perspective, is connected to relationships of power within the home care institution. Just as aides are used and abused by this system of care provision (as I outlined in chapter 1), so aides may use and abuse their clients. So the instances of theft, extortion, cheating in reporting hours, physical abuse of clients, and emotional abuse, while inexcusable, are the inevitable result of the power dynamic in home care (see chapter 5). Power manifests itself in a variety of ways and on a variety of levels.

Take the example of cheating in reporting one's hours. There is an increasing problem of home care aides recording hours when they are not actually working them: Some aides will double-book shifts with two home care agencies and report their hours to both companies. Or they will make deals with clients so that they do not show up for all scheduled shifts, yet they will report all scheduled hours to their home offices. Clients are often complicit in these arrangements for a variety of reasons: out of fear that their aide will be fired, out of fear that they will lose their home care hours if they complain about the aides, and out of a kinlike concern for the aide's personal life. For many reasons, these problems are arising as responses to the hierarchy and domination that inhere in the home care industry.

Such a Foucauldian read of home care should lead us to question whether home care really is a kinder, gentler, more humane form of care. While it may seem that this system of care provision better addresses the "whole person" in ways that institution-based care cannot, I have argued that home care often fails in this respect. Indeed, one could argue that rather than humanizing caretaking and bringing dependency needs back into the community, the institution of home care has served to further marginalize care by turning it into a shameful sign of one's incompetence and lack of independence.

In taking on a Foucauldian critique, the notion of progress becomes extremely problematic. This is because we can no longer see human history on a linear trajectory from ignorance to enlightenment, from subordination to freedom. On the contrary, Foucault reminds us that power is not to be overcome or eliminated; rather, it changes form, becomes internalized, and renders us agents in the practice of monitoring and disciplining ourselves and our bodies.

Yet I do not intend to take my Foucauldian critique that far. We *must* maintain some conception of progress, especially in areas like home care, where vulnerable people's lives are at stake. There are certainly better and worse ways of practicing home health care, and there are more and less negative means by which power is expressed. For example, physically abusing frail, elderly home care clients is arguably a much more negative expression of power relations than is the practice of cheating on one's home care hours. In constructing a philosophy of home care, then, I do not assume that power relations can be entirely overcome: but I do assume that a better system of home care is to be found outside a market-based model of care.

## Constructing a Rich Philosophy of Home Care

The preceding leads to the question: What should a philosophy of home care look like?[10] Below I will outline how it might be constructed, but first let me consider the issue of social justice. Whatever philosophy of home care that is adopted for the United States, it should have a social justice framework. Without such a framework, as we have seen, the philosophy may only serve the already powerful vested interests of corporate America. For this reason, as I will argue in chapter 3, we need a feminist ethics undergirding the philosophy, for feminist ethics is concerned with issues of social justice, particularly for women. Since home health care has been feminized, we need a focus on social justice that brings forth the exploitative structures that impact women in particular.

First, a philosophy of home care should be a philosophy of chronic care and not only in the ideological sense. Many commentators have claimed that home care is chronic care. True, what home care workers accomplish is meeting the chronic care needs of dependent citizens at home, but as I have argued, in practice home care is modeled on an acute care paradigm. Recall that Medicare limits on reimbursable care restrict services to patients who require skilled and intermittent care. A client must have a referring physician who has approved the course of treatment and identified the patient's skilled need. This means that the mundane needs created by aging and increasing fragility (the inability to get in and out of the tub without assistance, for example) are not included; *chronic care needs are excluded.*

Acute care has been the preferred model for organizing home care services because it avoids the messy, complex, and expensive chronic care demands that a chronic care model would have to address. These demands —including depression, poverty, ongoing and persistent illness or disability, nutritional deficiencies, and dementia, to name a few—are left for family members and poorly paid caretakers to deal with. A philosophy of home care that embraces chronic care would not treat these factors as side issues but would place them at the center of the care model. Chronic care requires a multifaceted approach to caretaking that acute care avoids. Clients should not have to wait for an acute episode in order to get the assistance of an aide at home; furthermore, there should be no skilled care requirement in order for them to receive services.

Second, a philosophy of home care should focus on caring about, not just caring for, clients: it should be a philosophy that encompasses the whole person. While caring for clients—offering physical care—is certainly an important part of home care service (since one's physical comfort is one aspect of the "whole person"), it is not all of it. There are both intrinsic and instrumental reasons for making caring about clients part of a philosophy of home care. Such care is intrinsically good because it is humane care, and because, whether or not a client flourishes when cared about, it is what makes each person unique in an otherwise impersonal system. "Caring about" is instrumentally good, too, because it often does lead to improved health and mental wellness. These are important instrumental goals in any system of health care.

If "caring about" is not an explicit part of home care's philosophy, then serious injustices result. Home care workers are allotted barely enough time to physically minister to clients such that, at the policy level, a mechanical approach is taken to caring, and clients are robbed of their particularity because they are treated as "things" to be moved, washed, and fed.

The philosophy of home care for which I am petitioning should also protect the vulnerable. As chapters 3 and 4 will argue, this includes both caretakers (paid and unpaid) and care recipients. Especially where issues of race and economic status arise (since aides are largely African American or Hispanic women of low economic status), we need to be mindful of practices and policies that further exploit them. Were we to take protection of the vulnerable seriously in the home care setting, we would need to move away from the market-driven, managed care model that currently guides home health care. For as chapter 1 indicates, the model itself assumes an ill-paid and/or unpaid female workforce.

Chapter 6 will consider in some detail the kind of changes required to make home care just. Here what I have offered is a prolegomena to the ethical practice of home care. When considering the philosophy of home health care, we must move beyond ideology and the current system of care provision to consider what it *could* be. While I reject the view that home care could ever be completely free of exploitation and relations of power, I do think that reform is possible and necessary.

The reform of home care practice is best achieved through a feminist ethics approach. Feminists have long treated issues of domination and subordination, care, justice, and relationships; and these are the very considerations that arise in the practice of home care. Let us now consider how a feminist ethical approach to home care can help to reform it.

# 3  Women's Care Work as a Subsidy to the State

In chapter 1, I argued that the home care system, in its current state, is morally lacking: It is founded on the broader system of managed care in the United States and is informed by the value of acute care that infuses health care practice at the macro level. Chapter 2 concerned the philosophy of home care and argued that there are competing and warring philosophies at the industrywide and home-based levels. In this chapter I will develop my argument that justice in home care requires the recognition of home care work as a social subsidy. Indeed, home care is not an area of narrow concern but involves broad cultural norms concerning the value of women's care work, the assignment to women of nurturing and caretaking, and their resulting economic and moral oppression.

## Home Caretaking as Subsidy

There are at least two possible responses to the system of home health care in its current incarnation: Work within the system to render it as efficient, as cost-effective, and as fair as possible to all parties involved, or opt for a different kind of system. In what follows I will petition for the latter, for the problems with our home health care system run too deep for mere reform. Since the very lives and livelihoods of some of our most vulnerable citizens are at stake, we require a system of home care delivery that is sensitive to their needs. So for those who require assistance with their activities of daily living (ADLS) and instrumental activities of daily living (IADLs), and for those who are called upon to offer the caretaking assistance, a re-vision of the home health care system is in order.

The informal provision of home health care is the foundation for home health services. Since patients are sent home from hospital "sicker and quicker," and formal home care services are generally provided for only 60 days after discharge from a hospital, this means that a great deal of caretaking falls upon families themselves. Home health services have also faced recent serious cutbacks, meaning that families must become ever more resourceful in finding means to provide care for their dependent family members. Usually this "resourcefulness" requires female family members to take leave from their paid employment in order to be available as familial caretakers; the result of such leaves can often be financially devastating to families, since women's employment is no longer supplemental and their income is no longer simply "pin money." Yet women's sense of responsibility for care of their family members results from the question of who else is going to do it. The inevitable answer is "no one."

To a large degree, economic privilege determines the degree to which families are strained by the demands of home care. For example, when working as a home health aide, I encountered two families dealing with remarkably similar situations. In both cases the clients with whom I was working, John and Bill, were teenagers who had been struck by cars as children. Both suffered severe brain damage. Their mothers were heads of household. But in one situation, John's mother had tapped her educational and community resources to sue the city for her son's accident; she had been awarded millions of dollars in compensation. Bill's mother had very little education, lacked any knowledge or understanding of her rights, had no community support in petitioning for them, and so never sought the legal compensation she was likely to be awarded. While neither boy received the amount of formal home care required, and both had to rely heavily on care by their mothers, John's care was much less onerous on his mother than was Bill's. Indeed, with the money from her lawsuit, John's mother was able to furnish him with a large, comfortable, fully equipped wheelchair-accessible home and van, and she had the economic ability to pay for extra attendant care to ease her own care burden. By contrast, Bill and his mother had no options available and remained in their low-income townhouse, where he was daily required to negotiate the narrow stairs lead-ing from the living room to his bedroom. After completing his toiletries, I would "spot" Bill as he came down the steep stairs. The shabby living room of their townhouse was so small that turning Bill around in his wheelchair had to be done slowly and with extreme care so that he didn't bump into furniture. His mother was a thin, frail woman who chain-smoked and wor-ried constantly. When Bill was not receiving his assistance through my home care office (which amounted to only twenty hours per week), his mother took on the care work herself. To this day I am powerfully struck by the situations of these two young men, their mothers, and the injustice of a care system that would allow and sustain such gross inequalities be-tween two very similar situations. Bill should not be daily placed at risk in a home hostile to his disabilities, and his mother, like John's, should have the resources to ease her care burden.

I cite these cases to highlight the way in which familial care burdens can be rendered heavy or light depending on the economic resources of the fam-ily unit. Where families are wealthier and able to hire caretakers, the care work can be better managed, and female family members can remain in full-time paid employment.[1] But ironically the working poor—those who can least afford to miss work—are most likely to lose paid work days or take sick leaves without pay in order to care for their family members. This is because the very fact of their poverty renders them incapable of seeking the assistance with caretaking that the wealthy are able to afford. In addi-tion, correlations between health and socioeconomic status mean that citi-zens who are economically the worst off are likely to suffer more serious health problems, thus rendering the working poor doubly burdened.

The caretaking required of ill or disabled family members is not a pri-vate problem for individual families. That American culture has, to this point, viewed illness and disability as private issues that must be dealt with by the individual and his/her family says more about our cultural values than about caretaking itself. It is neither inevitable nor necessary that we view home health care as a private, familial issue, for once we understand the degree to which caretaking is a social matter, we can consider social re-sponses to it.

Home health care is privatized in two ways: first, by understanding it as a problem for individual families and, second, by having the caretaking done almost entirely by women. Since women's caretaking has historically been associated with the so-called private sphere—that is, outside the bounds of public life—this association between women and caretaking has also resulted in the privatization of care work. Therefore, though the moth-ers in the above two cases may experience their caretaking demands differently (since John's mother can afford to hire an attendant to take on her care responsibilities), they both equally experience the *gendered* demands of caring.

Emily Abel addresses the demands of caretaking in women's lives as follows:

> When an older person with several surviving children becomes ill, relatives often designate a daughter or daughter-in-law, rather than a son or son-in-law, as the primary caregiver. The reigning ideology still holds that women are "natural" caregivers. Moreover, because women remain concentrated in low-paid and/or part-time jobs, families often view women's salaries as more easily dispensable and their work schedules as more flexible. (139)

What we need, then, is an ethic that is responsive to the particular issues raised by home care. Some feminist theorists have argued that an ethic of care is best-suited to this task. For example, Joan Tronto (1998) sees care as transformative and claims that we need to reassess the little social value placed on caring. In what follows I will highlight the care ethic as it has been identified by some feminist moral theorists; I will then consider its efficacy in attending to issues in home health care. Ultimately, as I will argue, an ethic of care alone fails as an ideal model on which to base this type of care.

### An Ethic of Care

Some feminist approaches to ethics are motivated by a singular moral perspective that is deemed characteristic of many women: an "ethic of care."[2] This ethic is characterized by an understanding of the individual as an interdependent, socially embedded being.[3] Such a conception of the individual goes against traditional accounts according to which we are independent subjects who relate to others in a detached manner. It also goes against traditional views about the nature of moral decision making. Traditional ethical theories demand that we make our moral decisions objectively and impartially (Kant, Mill). According to these theories, we must use our reasoning capacity and, as independent, rational agents, make our moral decisions based on objective considerations.

But feminist ethicists question the emphasis placed on objectivity, impartiality, reason, and independence. Instead, they argue that we are born into a web of relationships, beginning with our immediate families and extending later in life to include friends, significant others, colleagues, and so on. Our social embeddedness means that we are not the independent, objective, and impartial beings that traditional accounts have posited. On the contrary, we are *inter*dependent beings who need one another for emotional and physiological support. Furthermore, who we are—and what duties and rights we have with respect to others—is at least partly a function of the social roles we have taken on. For example, being a mother entails having certain obligations with respect to your child that are not shared by others. Finally, being socially embedded means that our moral understanding of ourselves and others is always contextually situated (e.g., a poor black woman will perceive certain aspects of social reality differently than a wealthy white man). Thus, feminist ethicists emphasize the contextual features of our lives over the abstract universal humanity that traditional ethicists claim is the ground of independence-securing rights, and they stress the importance of caring for others as the basis for our moral decision making.

Indeed, some care ethicists go even further in arguing that traditional approaches to ethics are actually immoral inasmuch as they ignore important contextual features of our lives. Moral theorist Nel Noddings argues that human relationships are based not on respect for individuals' abstract rights but rather on meeting the concrete needs of particular individuals. By demanding that we be detached, impartial agents, these traditional approaches deny our lived experiences and chasten us to ignore the particular features of our situations. Indeed, Noddings claims, "I shall reject ethics of principle as ambiguous and unstable. Wherever there is principle, there is implied exception and, too often, principles function to separate us from each other" (1984, 98). Some feminist ethicists claim that a "care" approach is a superior one because it takes seriously our caring relationships and the impact those relationships have on our moral decision making. Thus, as theorists like Sara Ruddick have argued, instead of focusing on contractual human relationships we ought rather to take the mother-child relationship as paradigmatic of all human relationships, since this relationship is at least as representative of human interactions as the contractual view.

Carol Gilligan was first to identify an ethic of care that undergirds women's lives and provides them with a moral identity different from men's. Furthermore, her work allowed women to embrace the ethic of care, since it was found to be no less justified than (and thus, not inferior to) the "justice" perspective—or focus on principles, objectivity, and impartiality that mark the traditional, moral approach into which men are socialized.[4] The ethic of care was liberatory for women in that it embraced women's particular ways of "doing" moral reasoning and allowed for the inclusion of more personal considerations in moral theory.[5] Rather than working from the level of abstract moral theories to determine what should be done in specific circumstances, the ethic of care begins with the particular features of one's own personal relationships with others.

The care ethic has been discussed by a variety of feminist moral theorists, and while some have been critical of it, most embrace its underlying premise that human beings are interdependent beings in relationships of care.[6] As Gilligan states,

> As a framework for moral decision, care is grounded in the assumption reflected in a view of action as responsive and, therefore, as arising in relationship rather than the view of action as emanating from within the self and, therefore, "self governed." Seen as responsive, the self is by definition connected to others, responding to perceptions, interpreting events, and governed by the organizing tendencies of human interaction and human language. (1987, 24)

Thus, while not unproblematic, an ethic of care results in a distinctly nontraditional way of conceiving moral reasoning.

Unfortunately, this has not prevented actual practices of caring from serving traditional patriarchy. This is nowhere more evident that in the appeals to home care as a preferential care paradigm, where women's willingness as caring persons to provide free and/or cheap labor is taken for granted. For example, the U.S. government holds the nuclear family responsible for the care of the elderly by treating the family as a sphere of privacy immune to public intervention. Care of the elderly falls squarely on female members of the household, whose labor has traditionally been confined to domestic caregiving. As Alan Walker claims, this means that "women and families continue to bear the social costs of dependency [while] the privatisation of family life protects 'normal' inequalities between family members" (121).

Feminist critics of home care have rightly objected to the government's reliance on women in upholding the cost-effectiveness of home care programs.[7] But what these critics often ignore is the underlying ethical basis for this exploitation: the systemic perversion of care ethics. Instead of enhancing the proper caring nature of all relationships, this ethic functions by legitimizing as "natural" the exploitation of women's domestic work. Let us consider in detail how women's care work is naturalized by the system.

### Essentializing Care Ethics

Whenever women's care work is viewed as "naturally feminine," an ethic of care is naturalized. To be sure, home health care is not the only arena in which care work is naturalized as feminine. Other instances include child-rearing, care for people with mental disabilities, nursing, primary school teaching, day care, and elder care. Indeed, since home care is modeled on these precedents, it should come as no surprise that it shares their patriarchal assumptions.[8]

Caring is tied not only to women but to the private sphere where intimate relationships flourish. This is primarily the sphere of the home and family: Since women have historically been linked to the private sphere of the home, the task of caring "naturally" devolves upon them. Women internalize the caring mentality to such a degree that, if they are accused of not caring enough, they feel guilty.

Remarking on this syndrome, Jean Grimshaw notes that while an ethic of care should not render women responsible for all care work, its patriarchal distortion has that effect.

> What does care for children entail, for example? Is it a failure of care not to be available on demand to one's child twenty-four hours a day for the first five years of their lives? . . . Is it a failure of care to insist on a holiday alone away from one's elderly parents? . . . Women in particular are often prone to feelings of guilt if they try to seize a bit of space, time or privacy for themselves, away from other people. They are especially vulnerable to charges of not-caring, since they are so often seen as defined by their caring role and capacities. (217)

Furthermore, because in the caring feminine psyche women often find it difficult caring for themselves, the moral boundaries between self and other become blurred. This results in a difficulty in demanding care, for women tend to identify their good as bound up with that of the others who are dependent upon them; hence, caring for others may result in dangerous forms of self-abnegation or altruism.

Bonnelle Lewis Strickling emphasizes that self-abnegation—denial of oneself—has long been held a feminine virtue. She identifies two forms: moral and metaphysical/epistemological. Strickling points out that the former requires setting aside the things one values for the sake of others; the latter, by contrast, involves losing oneself in these others. Although all human beings are encouraged to practice a modest degree of moral self-abnegation (morality, after all, involves entering into the worldview of another), it is only women who are expected to practice metaphysical/epistemological self-abnegation, or the total forsaking of one's self. And, says Strickling, the result is a failure to develop one's own sense of self, which may cause enormous resentment or anger on the part of the self-abnegator (190, 197). Her concerns are thus closely linked to home care as practiced by both female family members and paid female caregivers: In both instances, women who care for others often develop a weak sense of self, which leads to despair, resentment, and anger on the part of the caregiver.

Consider, for example, the large amounts of personal, unpaid time that women are expected to put toward care for others. As a home care aide, I often found myself placed in the difficult situation of choosing between finishing my shifts on time (and thus serving my own needs) or staying beyond my paid hours in order to avoid abandoning my clients. One particular elderly client would beg me to stay longer every time I visited her. Since she was living alone, afraid of the dark, and suffering from mild dementia, I often found myself staying several hours beyond my scheduled shift, resenting my employer for putting me in this situation and feeling guilty for feeling resentment.[9]

The inclusiveness of women's moral boundaries and the naturalizing feminization of the ethic of care thus results in an unhappy situation for female caregivers, paid and unpaid. Caregivers often end up putting in far more time than they can afford, losing a clear sense of where their needs start and where the needs of those who are dependent on them end, and feeling frustrated, forsaken, and desperate. These aspects of home health care—its foundations in women's exploitation and the co-optation of women's sense of responsibility for others—renders it unethical. The question then becomes whether home health care has the potential to be less exploitative and alienating for the caregiver.

In what follows I will argue that home care can be rendered less exploitative and alienating, but only if we address the practice from a self-consciously feminist perspective.[10] Furthermore, the feminist perspective we adopt, though borrowing elements from an ethic of care, must have an explicit social and political agenda.[11] While an ethic of care identifies a legitimate moral perspective that derives from our relational selves,[12] it lacks a social and political component that raises questions such as Who does the caring? At what cost? What presuppositions and theoretical assumptions undergird the conception and practice of home care? This social and political critique, however, cannot rest with feminist critics alone; it must be a focal concern for all those involved in home health care, from government officials and public policymakers to home care supervisors and fieldworkers.

### Politicizing Care Ethics

In her work, Susan Sherwin critiques systems of health care from such a politicized care perspective. She identifies the ethic of care as a "feminine" ethic and distinguishes it from "the explicitly political perspective of feminism, where the oppression of women is seen to be morally and politically unacceptable" (35). On her view, while we must respect the unique moral perspective of women, we must also ensure justice by examining the oppressive practices by which women are subordinated. In short, this requires establishing moral criteria for determining when to offer and when to withhold care, an element of caring that is not addressed by care ethicists like Noddings.

Sherwin applies her self-consciously feminist approach to bioethics and health care. She indicates that both have been conceived, discussed, and practiced so as to serve an agenda that marginalizes and subordinates women and other historically oppressed groups. I think Sherwin is right and that her general critique of bioethics and health care applies to the practice of home health care specifically. Home health care is infused with the same system of values, the same language, and the same norms that drive our health care systems generally.[13]

Helga Kuhse is equally critical of an ethic of care that lacks a social and political basis. In her work on nursing ethics, Kuhse argues that without being tempered by concerns for justice, a nursing ethic of care is ultimately conservative and oppressive for women. This nursing ethic has been identified as a way of distinguishing the nurse's focus on caring from medicine's concern with curing. By embracing an ethic of care, some nursing theorists have argued, nurses can identify an ethic that is unique to the practice of nursing: that is, caring and patient advocacy. Yet the nursing profession is still dominated by women, so appealing to a nursing ethic of care can be politically dangerous. It robs nurses of the moral grounds to petition for fair wages, to strike, to speak out when they are treated unjustly by patients, and to resist being overburdened by huge patient loads. So, as Kuhse rightly argues, "Care is . . . a necessary but not a sufficient condition for an ethics that will serve patients and nurses well. An adequate ethics needs impartiality or justice as well as care" (145).

Finally, Barbara Houston also cautions feminists against overenthusiastically embracing an ethic of care. While Houston does not denigrate the virtuous activities of caretaking, nurturing, and "sustaining the growth of other moral subjects" (239), she questions the unqualified reclamation of "womanly virtues."

Ways of life produced by a system of interlocking barriers that serve to limit women's choices and options should be addressed suspiciously. For example, the uncritical embracing of a feminine care ethic glosses over the history of women's nurturance and care work, in which (as Strickling points out) women give freely while expecting nothing in return. As Houston argues, there are dangers in rescuing "womanly" virtues, primarily the dangers of gender essentialism, and glorifying women's oppression (256).

Thus, we need a blend of a partialist advocacy for special moral attachments and responsibilities and an impartialist emphasis on principled moral theorizing that stresses objectivity, universalizability, and justice. Without regard for impartialist concerns, feminists cannot petition for the rights of female caregivers. Indeed, I am critical of home health care precisely because it has been guided entirely by an ethic of care, without sufficient concern for justice.

Let us consider a *politicized* feminist ethical critique of home health care and the difference effected by it. A feminist ethic requires us to deconstruct the normative assumptions that undergird home health care, for example, assumptions about the desirability of remaining in one's own home, the importance of autonomy, and the value of independence, as well as norms surrounding "women's work." These are some of the normative assumptions that feminist moral theorists have been resisting.

### Autonomy and Independence

The popularity of home health care derives, at least in part, from our cultural preoccupation with autonomy and independence. Feminist moral theorists have been critical of this focus, especially in the realm of health care. Autonomy is a formative notion on which North American culture and our system of health care delivery is largely based. Indeed, it has become the foundational principle of health care.[14] Consider, for example, the "Patient Bill of Rights" that hangs above virtually every hospital admissions desk across the country. The visible posting of this bill serves to indicate the hospital's serious commitment to patient autonomy and reassure patients that their autonomy will be respected. Such a preoccupation with autonomy belies our tragic awareness that we ultimately lack governance over aging, illness, disability, suffering, and death. To admit this lack of autonomy is to recognize that the human condition is beyond our control; to relinquish autonomy is to acknowledge our existence in vulnerable bodies.

Furthermore, this preoccupation with autonomy relates to independence, for a citizen's independence and her ability to live independently of others is symbolic of her autonomy. It is no small wonder, then, that most individuals prefer to be cared for at home, where their surroundings are familiar and comforting and where their return to their homes further symbolizes their independence and autonomy. Dependency has been associated with weakness, incapacity, neediness, and a lack of dignity; and insofar as individuals are able to resist dependency, they are able to maintain their dignity and self-respect. If home care assists individuals in the realization of these goods, then it is all the more culturally desirable.

On many occasions during my tenure as a home care aide, I witnessed care receivers' attempts to maintain their autonomy and independence. They did this in small but meaningful ways. For example, in some cases they instructed me on how to complete tasks around their homes: the "correct" way to wash laundry, do dishes, clean the bathroom, and fold clothing. By overseeing my visits to their homes, they were able to maintain control over their home environments and ensure that tasks were completed as *they* would do them. Furthermore, this enabled them to relate to others as autonomous, independent equals (for example, casually stating in conversation that "my aide is such a good little worker," much as others speak of their housekeepers). While I found my clients' attempts to control my services sometimes annoying and insulting, their need to assert their independence and autonomy was understandable in a culture that hyper-values those qualities.

Feminist moral theorists do not denigrate the importance of autonomy. On the contrary, given its historical denial to women, they are concerned with protecting and preserving it. But they do not treat autonomy as the only, or most important, social value, since other values such as equality or reciprocity are also at risk. Feminists query why furthering the autonomy of the client has to involve jeopardizing (or relinquishing) the autonomy of the caregiver. Thus, a politicized feminist ethic, though valuing autonomy, questions its primacy, especially insofar as it is traceable to a philosophical history that valorizes objectivity and impartiality. Furthermore, as chapter 4 will indicate, feminists support a concept of relational autonomy that differs from traditional conceptions of it.

The moral basis for home health care is therefore questionable, for from a feminist perspective, the individual's desire to maintain her autonomy and independence (or, at least, the semblance of them) is not benign. If autonomy and independence are synonymous with the good, and dependency and relationality are synonymous with the bad, then it is unsurprising that home care is preferred over institutional care.

### Politicizing Dependency and Dependency Workers

A second critique of home health care returns to my previous assertion that caregiving devolves upon women because their caregiving is naturalized. Home health care services are required in our current social context given that home is where individuals clearly want to be.[15] Since home care is rooted in the private sphere of the home, and care work historically has been construed as "women's work," the provision of home care has fallen almost exclusively on women, both as unpaid family caregivers and as formal, paid caregivers. From a feminist politicized ethical perspective, however, the problem is not only that women have primarily been responsible for care for dependents. It is that theories of justice have allowed women to unfairly and unequally shoulder the burden of care. Justice for female caregivers cannot be achieved if theories of justice do not account for this basic inequality. I think that theories of justice can address the unfair burden of women's care work, but so far they have failed to do so.

Eva Kittay has addressed the question of justice for female caregivers—what she calls "dependency workers"—from the liberal tradition in ethics. Using John Rawls's theory of justice (1971) as her starting point, Kittay argues that dependent persons and dependency workers must be given special consideration in order to be included in the community of equal citizens. She criticizes Rawls for defining "the political" in terms set out by traditional political philosophies that ignore responsibility for dependents. Rawls, like his predecessors, assumes that dependency responsibility belongs to citizens' private lives, not the realm of public life. Yet, as Kittay asserts, dependency is a political issue, and care is one of the most basic elements of a flourishing society (1997, 220).

Thus, the problem with liberal theorists like Rawls is his focus on political equality, that is, the focus on the public realm where equality and justice between heads of households is the main concern. Rawls never addresses the question of equality and justice *within* the family (the private sphere). Rawls's theory does not consider justice for dependency workers, like home health aides or family caretakers, because they do not inhabit the public realm where political equality is addressed.[16] Yet, as Kittay indicates, dependency "is a matter for us all in our lives as social beings" (1997, 221). To be sure, dependence and dependency work are features of all our lives. We are born dependent and, with aging and the possibility of disablement, we are likely to return to a state of dependency. But barring this contingency, we are all likely to care for dependents at some point in our lives, whether it be our children, partners, siblings, or elderly parents.

Kittay addresses the problem of reciprocity for dependency workers by invoking "doulia," a concept she takes from the practice of some traditional cultures where a doula is assigned to assist caregivers. For example, a doula might assist a new mother in caring for herself while she is caring for her infant; in short, doulas are part of a system of nested dependencies.[17] As Kittay states,

> Extending the notion of the service performed by the doula, let us use the term "doulia" to refer to an arrangement by which service is passed on so that those who become needy by virtue of tending to those in need can be cared for as well. Doulia is part of an ethic that is captured in the collo-

quial phrase "What goes around comes around." . . . We can state the principle of doulia: *Just as we have required care to survive and thrive, so we need to provide conditions that allow others—including those who do the work of caring—to receive the care they need to survive and thrive.* (1997, 233)

Thus, as she indicates, dependence (and dependency work) affect our status as equal citizens when their burdens are unequally shouldered. Any theory of justice that sets them aside as private concerns fails to address core issues concerning the structure of society. A theory of justice, as Kittay argues, must concern itself with who does the care work, the effects of that work on the citizen's social and political equality, and the distribution of dependency work.

That home care (and all other forms of caretaking) naturally devolves upon women, then, is a core issue for any theory of justice. Rawls claims that a well-ordered society is one that is pluralistic, in which "the public agreement on questions of political and social justice supports ties of civic friendship and secures the bonds of association" (1980, 520). But, as Kittay indicates, more central here are the bonds of caregiving and personal relationship that undergird the very possibility for "civic friendship" and "the bonds of association." Furthermore, as Kittay claims, any decent society must provide all members with a basis for self-respect by publicly acknowledging care as a basic good. Such care must be provided in a way that is fair, comprehensive, and inclusive (1997, 235).

Disability theorist Mary Mahowald highlights the dismissive and disrespectful treatment to which dependency workers are vulnerable, treatment which may deny caregivers their self-respect. She observes the dismissive social treatment of personal attendants caring for persons with disabilities, indicating their treatment as *things* rather than persons. Here Mahowald substantiates Kittay's claim that dependency work, in our current social milieu, may erode the workers' self-respect; indeed, any home care worker who has been ignored by the home care receiver's visiting friends or family—as if she were simply not there—knows of this experience. We thus need a good dose of justice mixed with care in the home care setting in order to ensure that home caregivers (and receivers) have respect (and self-respect) and that the care work is shared equally by all members of society.

Home health care, then, is not beyond the purview of justice. Although it takes place in the so-called private realm of the home and family, its practice has serious implications for a just and well-ordered society. In its current manifestation, home care is unjust, for it is based on a devaluing of the home care worker and her freedom and on a poorly paid and unpaid female workforce whose political equality is compromised. And though some feminists have indicted governments and home care agencies for exploiting women's care work, they have failed to place this exploitation within the framework of a theory of justice. Indeed, as Holstein claims, the adage "the personal is political" has particular relevance for home health care, since one major task suggested by a feminist politicized ethic is to ensure support and assistance for women (including family members) who are caregiving at great risk, both personally and economically (239).

### Reconciling Justice with Care

Martha Fineman has argued:

> If infants or ill persons are not cared for, nurtured, nourished, and perhaps loved, they will perish. We can say, therefore, that they owe an individual debt to their individual caretakers. But the obligation is not theirs alone— nor is their obligation confined only to their own caretakers. A sense of social justice demands a broader sense of obligation. Without aggregate caretaking, there could be no society, so we might say that it is caretaking labor that produces and reproduces society. Caretaking labor provides the citizens, the workers, the voters, the consumers, the students, and others who populate society and its institutions. The uncompensated labor of caretakers is an unrecognized subsidy, not only to individuals who directly receive it, but more significantly, to the entire society. (19)

By recognizing the free and cheap labor provided by female home caretakers, and the state's reliance on such care as basic to the well-being of society, we can begin to glean the import of such caretaking work. Imagine what would happen if family caretakers and paid home care aides went on strike, if their "nonproductive" labor of bathing, feeding, dressing, providing medications, making beds, doing laundry, buying groceries, and making meals ceased overnight. Such a scenario is unthinkable—both because we cannot imagine families refusing to care for (and about) their loved ones in this way, and because there would be nobody to take up the slack. In short, there are no "scabs" in the caretaking arena. Arguably, under such conditions, society would virtually shut down, and life would, as Thomas Hobbes put it, become "solitary, poor, nasty, brutish, and short" (186).

The notion of women's caretaking as a subsidy to the state is radical and has not been taken up as a serious proposal because of the dominance of right-wing ideology. Indeed, caretaking remains a marginalized political consideration because conservative ideology upholds a hierarchical and patriarchal vision of it as a private affair to be addressed by poorly paid or unpaid women in families with male heads of household (McCluskey, 118). Again, the "private sphere" ideology rears its ugly head.

Beyond these ideologies, however, lies the pitting of efficiency against justice and the notion that recognizing and remunerating home caretaking is both inefficient and dangerous. Efficiency involves promoting overall economic gain, or maximizing aggregate gains, while justice entails moving resources around to benefit particular individuals or groups. As Martha McCluskey points out, dominant economic theory privileges efficiency over justice, and instructs that redistributive policies (like paid home caretaking) are a bad idea because they have negative consequences for all. For example, redistributing resources to subsidize family caretaking and to better pay home care aides may be a good short-term approach. But in the long run, such a redistribution will result in overall economic hardship that harms everyone, including those who were supposed to benefit from the redistribution. Eventually monies will dry up, as the state cannot sustain such subsidies to caretakers on a long-term basis (123).

But, as McCluskey states, "the ostensibly neutral idea of 'efficiency' always incorporates assumptions about whose particular interests are taken as the standard for determining society's well-being. Feminists should ask the question: efficient for whom, according to what standard?" (127). Thus, objections to the redistribution of social goods to pay home caretakers already assumes a certain definition of "efficiency" (as economic growth) and an understanding of caretakers' interests as "private." Rather than resting on good arguments, the claim that public support of capital, not caretaking, will best serve all citizens is resting on "ideological faith" (131). Indeed, there is no good economic evidence for the idea that capital growth best serves most citizens. Economic growth notoriously serves only the wealthiest members of society and tends to widen the income gap between rich and poor. As McCluskey indicates, the economic booms that supposedly benefited all in the 1980s and 1990s served only to improve the situation of the rich: "The top one percent of wealth holders received sixty-two percent of the total gain in marketable wealth between 1983 and 1989, while the 'bottom' eighty percent of Americans received only one percent of this growth" (132). "Efficiency" objections to paid family caretaking and raises in payments to home health aides are thus groundless when one scrutinizes how efficiency gets defined and who gets to define it.[18]

Fineman's reconceptualization of women's caretaking work as a subsidy to the state must be taken seriously if we truly care about subordinated members of society. For the sake of both care recipients and caretakers, we must take seriously the notion that something is owed, on a social level, to women who are unpaid or underpaid for their caretaking work. Indeed, as I have indicated, in doing such work women risk a great deal.

The work of feminists like Fineman and Kittay has been essential to bringing a caretaking agenda to our political discourse. These theorists do an excellent job of highlighting the absolute necessity to our social and political lives of formal and informal caretaking. But what Fineman and Kittay have not sufficiently addressed is the importance of *paid* caretakers and how responsibility is constructed such that caretakers as employees are also at risk. If we focus too closely on families in connection to care, we will miss the broader issue of paid caretakers (like home care aides) and the ways in which paid and unpaid caretakers are connected. Let us now focus on the risks associated with home care work for paid caretakers and the ways in which familial caretaking issues are linked to the injustices faced by these formal, paid employees.

We cannot approach a public solution to ethical problems in home health care without considering all affected parties. Home health aides are the lowest paid of any workers in the caretaking industry, including nursing home aides, who are notoriously badly paid. Home health care is premised on the free and cheap care provided by female family members and paid (mostly female) caretakers; indeed, some critics have argued that wages for home health aides are necessarily low in order to keep home care affordable. But if one adds in the amount of unpaid hours that aides put in (because they often stay to comfort clients long past their scheduled hours), their lack of benefits (including social security, paid vacation, sick leave, maternity leave, and health insurance), and their unpaid travel time between clients' homes, then the wages are worse than one might initially think. Add to this the emotionally taxing labor that they perform, since paid caretakers are providing emotional care, and not just physical care, for their clients, and one gets an even better sense of why the home care industry suffers from recruitment and retention problems with its workforce.

Home care aides lack the professional status that affords them recognition and respect for their work. Often referred to as "para-professional" or "nonprofessional" work, this lack of professional status is arguably linked to their low remuneration for difficult and heavy toil.[19] With reference to Michael Bayles's work on professionalism, Kittay (1999, 38–39) indicates the earmarks of a profession, including (1) extensive training, (2) training that involves a large intellectual element, and (3) work that provides an important service to the community. Beyond these main three elements, there are usually also processes of certification, an organization of members, and a considerable degree of autonomy. So physicians, for example, spend upwards of ten years in medical school and residency training; they must prove themselves intellectually to enter into the profession of medicine; and they provide an essential service to society. Physicians must pass strict certification requirements and usually belong to professional groups like the American Medical Association (AMA). Finally, physicians have had considerable autonomy in carrying out their work—at least, prior to the genesis of managed care.

Home care aides, by contrast, are considered nonprofessional because training is minimal (most training programs for home care aides last only about a week), they perform physical, rather than mental, labor, and the service they provide is not highly socially valued.[20] Home care aides have no guild or association through which they are organized. Furthermore, as Kittay also recognizes, work of professional status is functionally specific, while that of workers like home care aides is functionally diffuse. Physicians and lawyers are trained to do a particular kind of task. They intervene, and when their intervention is complete, they step away. By contrast, home care aides perform a diffuse and varied number of tasks that include physical, emotional, and psychological care. The work is repetitive and sometimes unending (1999, 41).

Home care aides, then, suffer from a cluster of related problems: They are poorly paid, they lack benefits, and they are viewed as nonprofessionals. Indeed, it is difficult to determine whether aides are poorly paid and, as a result, are not viewed as professionals, or whether they are poorly paid because they are not so viewed. What we do know, however, is that home care aides are almost always women and that the low pay is justified because they are performing "women's work," work that is understood as a "labor of love" rather than as necessary employment to make ends meet.

Clearly, gender, economic, and class issues arise in considerations of home health care. But as I mentioned in chapter 1, race is also an important element in any ethical examination of this practice. The largest proportion of home care aides are Hispanic and African American women; sometimes they do not speak English, and usually they are not well educated or trained in skilled work. Home care agencies, then, constitute a new job ghetto, where these women are put to work for very little money. Alternatively, families that can afford to pay out of pocket for assistance with home health needs often hire minority women because they are cheap and (it is believed) acquiescent employees.

Thus, we should not turn solely to the family to locate the ethical and political problems with home health care, for these problems are also situated outside the family unit, involving paid employees who face the same kinds of hardships as family caretakers or worse. Sometimes families themselves may exacerbate the ill treatment of caretakers; in addition to this, however, the more we focus on caretaking in the family context, the more I think we will continue to see it as a private, familial matter.

While Fineman and Kittay certainly *intend* their feminist critiques to include paid caretakers, they do not adequately incorporate the particular problems faced by paid, frontline workers like home care aides. While both family and paid caretakers suffer the diminished status of care work, and both experience the gendered burden of caring, paid caretakers face additional employment-related issues that are overlooked unless we expressly address paid caretaking.[21]

For example, consider what home health aides are being paid to do. By many accounts, formal caretakers are paid for doing physical, unskilled labor that requires no special talent. It is true that almost anyone can do the simple chores that home care aides are assigned, such as changing bedding, bathing bodies, and feeding mouths. But if the physical labor is really all that a home care aide's job is about, then one could just as well be caring for an animal as for a human being.[22] Chapter 2 treats the philosophies of home care and how we should understand the home care aide's job. Briefly put, reducing the work to physical labor violates the dignity and self-respect of both caretaker and care recipient, since it is akin to viewing care for dependents as caring for "things," and it robs home care aides of their own intuition that they may be skilled caretakers who have a special talent for working with others. Beyond this, such a reductionist reading of the home care aide's work denies the truth of the matter—that when persons are hired, they are hired for emotional and psychological support of the client, not just to service physical needs.

As an ex–home care aide, I can name dozens of situations where my work involved much more emotional and psychological than physical care of my charges. One client, Daniel, was assigned four hours of home care a week; and although I was sent to do housekeeping chores while he recuperated from surgery—what he called a "snip and clip" job to remove a cancer spot on his lung—I spent most of my time playing cribbage with him. Daniel was lonely (he lived alone in a trailer park), and the cancer scare shook him up such that he needed companionship more than he needed his bed made. In another instance, I was assigned to an elderly woman who was placed in the psychiatric unit of a nursing home. The woman was befuddled but conscious enough of her surroundings to be afraid of them. I was sent in to help her to the bathroom and assist with meals; I spent most of my time rubbing her back and trying to comfort and calm her down. Yet another elderly woman was in the early stages of Alzheimer's disease and was no longer competent to get her own meals and prepare herself for bed. I was there from 4 to 7 P.M. to make sure she ate dinner, had a bath, and got safely into bed. But again I found that the biggest part of my work with Marion involved comforting her. She would become anxious and agitated as night fell; as the time for my departure neared, she would start to moan, cry, and beg me to stay. Marion had lost her husband just months earlier and felt completely at sea. I believe to this day that our conversations did much more for her than my physical ministrations, for during the time that I was caring for her she finally agreed to move to an assisted living site. Her decision to move followed months of our client-aide relationship, where we repeatedly discussed the pros and cons of nursing home life.

My tenure as a home care aide involved both good and bad experiences, but the best of my work came from the above-cited relationships with my clients. I was good at my job: not just good at bathing people (though some skill is involved when a client with dementia refuses to get in the bathtub) but at doing the necessary emotional and psychological care. Those who understand the work of a home care aide as reducible to physical labor, then, either do not have family members who have ever required care, have never required care themselves, or completely lack moral imagination.

Across the board, home care aides list their personal connections with clients as the most fulfilling aspect of their work.[23] Thus, understanding the home care aide's job as washing bodies and feeding mouths not only minimizes the true breadth of her work, but is devastating to those aides who understand themselves in a more relational sense, as helping to make clients feel as much as possible like whole persons, and as treating them accordingly. We should no more treat home care aides as minions who perform physical tasks than we should view physicians as plumbers who unclog blocked arteries and repair heart valves.[24]

### Making Home Health Care Just

Since home health care is rooted in the exploitation of women's care work, I argue that its practice is inherently unjust. It is not simply that we need to pay home care workers more or ensure their receipt of benefits like health care insurance or sick leave; we need a much more radical approach if we are to make it a just and ethical practice. What we require, then, is no less than a complete rethinking of some of our commonly held tenets, such as the belief that caretaking issues are private matters to be taken up by individual families. As long as we retain this belief on the social level, the state will continue to piggyback on the free and low-cost care provided by women. And since the very premise of home care is built on our cultural support of the private/public split, no less than sweeping changes—both practical and ideological—will do.

On the level of ideological change, we need to alter our thinking regarding caretaking as women's work, and we need to see care as fundamental to the well-being and well-functioning of our society. These are points for which I have been arguing throughout the last three chapters; ones that have been vigorously and effectively argued by feminists like Martha Fineman, Eva Kittay, Joan Tronto, Martha Holstein, and Martha Minow. But there are also ideological changes to our ways of thinking about home care aides in particular that require change. Primarily, we need to rethink our conception of home care aides as "nonprofessional" or "para-professional" workers whose job is solely the physical maintenance of people in their homes.

Home care employment should take an entirely different direction if the industry is to secure a stable, satisfied, and enduring workforce. We will never pay home care workers—or family caretakers—a decent wage so long as we understand home care from a voluntaristic model. Few family members "volunteer" to care for ill and frail family members; rather, necessity, strong familial ties, and a sense of moral obligation dictate that care be offered. And in the case of paid caretakers, while more than mercenary considerations lead one into work as a home care aide, one should not be *penalized* for caring about one's clients by being badly paid for the work.

The value of philosophical imagination cannot be overstated here: We need to be able to "imagine ourselves otherwise"[25] in order to achieve anything. In applying our imaginative philosophical powers, we can ask ourselves: *What would home care look like if what founded it was a conception of citizens as persons involved in relationships of care?* This conception of citizenship (as suggested by Joan Tronto) is far more inclusive because all of us are either in need of care or are providing care for others. Caring practice is what makes us part of a community, a political system, and an economic system. So if we imagine citizens as first and foremost carers, we can imagine an entirely different system of political participation. By being more inclusive, this may positively affect how we understand who can and should participate in the formation of care policies.

Ultimately I want to deflect attention away from the debate between those who want to entirely socialize and publicize women's care work and those who want to individualize the care needs of citizens and keep them within the private realm. Neither response is appropriate. Responses to the care needs of citizens cannot come from just the government or just from families and their paid, private caretakers. They cannot come from the government alone because the state often fails in understanding the real needs of dependent persons. Because it is impersonal, economically oriented, and acontextual, we cannot simply invoke state responsibility and the need for state intervention without calling for a community response to caretaking needs. Furthermore, the most radical and effective efforts at social change often occur at the level of grassroots civic organizations that are attached to particular communities. In other words, we will need both state oversight of home care and local organizing surrounding its practice in order to achieve an effective, just, and caring version of home care.

### Conclusion: Care and Justice for Home Care Workers

As I have indicated, an ethic of care, though desirable in its focus on interdependence, relationships, nurturing, and care, fails to address the social and political injustices that render home health care unethical. While the parochialism of this care ethic is well suited to home health care, since it is practiced within the familial, private realm, a feminist ethic requires a further political agenda that takes home health care *beyond* parochialism. As Kuhse, Kittay, and others argue, those who work in nursing, elder, day, and home care need justice as well as care to guide their professions.

An example of the melding of care and justice is the recent unionization of home care workers in the United States. Seventy-five thousand workers in Los Angeles County voted to join the Service Employees International Union (SEIU) in an attempt to organize some of the nation's lowest paid workers. Along with unionization comes the hope that home care workers will increase their poverty-line wages and ensure better benefits and protection. The move to unionize follows the discovery that "people caring for animals at the Los Angeles Zoo earned three times as much as home-care workers" and that "you could triple [home care workers'] wages and still save money."[26] Unionization serves not only home care workers but also care receivers, since another union goal is to significantly lower the high turnover rate among home care workers. The home care industry has the largest turnover rate of all service industries—between 40 and 70 percent—and many caregivers leave jobs they like because of financial need. By having a stable, unionized home care workforce, we can ensure justice for workers and improve care for clients, since stable, long-term home care relationships between aide and client improve the effectiveness of the care. I will say more about this in chapter 6.

Furthermore, by melding care with justice we identify not only responsibilities of the worker but responsibilities *to* the worker. As Robyn Stone and Yoshiko Yamada suggest, previous accounts of home health care have focused on "frontline" long-term care workers' responsibilities to care recipients without demanding reciprocity. Yet, as Stone and Yamada argue, these workers

> have rights as well as responsibilities, and the ethical concerns regarding their status and treatment in the workplace and in society must be recog-

nized. What is more . . . nursing home and home care aides are moral
agents, and the ethical soul-searching should not be left to the workers'
superiors, as some have argued.[27]

I experienced this need in my own home care work for an ethic that addresses workers' status and treatment in the workplace. On several different occasions I was harassed, sometimes sexually. The harassment went
unrecognized by others, including my superiors, because it took place in the
privacy of the care receivers' homes; in any case, I felt so humiliated and de-
graded that I lacked the courage to complain. But my failure to report these
incidences also related to the fact that little could be done to protect workers. If I had complained, I might have been transferred out of those homes,
but another aide would surely have taken my place. I was reluctant to allow
the abuse to be passed on to another vulnerable female. And given the high
turnover rate, there were never enough workers to meet client demands, so
care coordinators were often angered by "problem" workers who made
their coordinating role more difficult. Focusing on the responsibilities of
caretakers to care receivers clearly does not address such injustices that
frontline caretakers experience at the hands of the home care industry.

But a feminist ethical analysis of home health care must not overlook
the other group of women who are moral subjects of concern: the many elderly females who receive care. While feminists have been critical of home
as a site for health care, they have often overlooked the elderly women who
may benefit from it. Thus, any justice-based or care-based account of home
care must consider it from the perspective of all those affected, especially
the marginalized group of elderly women who rely on it. The next chapter
will balance the interests of female home caretakers against those of the
cared-for. I will explore feminist ethical concerns regarding the treatment of
elderly women in our society and suggest that we should equally weigh the
needs of elderly female care recipients when considering the ethics of home
health care. There seems to be a tension for feminists between securing justice for home caretakers and avoiding the further marginalization and subordination of home care recipients. While I ultimately argue that the
interests of these two parties are connected, we must take care not to reduce
the ethics of home health care to concerns for the caretakers alone. Indeed,
as we will see, elderly female care recipients are also caretakers themselves,
so any theory of justice in home health care must also seek justice for them.

# 4 | Caring about the Cared-For

The previous three chapters have considered ethical issues in home health care with regard to caretakers. As I have argued, home health care is founded on the free and low-cost care labor provided by women. Ideologies that connect family with the private sphere, and that treat home care issues as private family matters, result in the depoliticization of its practice. Yet if we consider care as a universal, basic need for all citizens, then we can better understand caretaking as a social/political issue, not just a private one. This leads us to consider what respect and justice require in connection to home care workers and family caretakers. Clearly, we can and should do more to ensure that the care work done by these citizens is better remunerated, recognized, and valued.

One may think that by addressing justice issues for caretakers one has addressed the most pressing ethical issues in home health care. This is not the case, however. Addressing caretakers, while important, is a prolegomena to ethical issues in home care. The perspectives of care recipients are also central to any treatment of ethics and home health care, and from a feminist ethics approach, failing to include the perspectives of the cared-for may signal unsavory patterns of domination and subordination that require further investigation.

In this chapter I will balance the interests of caretakers against those of the cared-for. Since most home care recipients are elderly women, I will focus on this group, though my account is intended to be inclusive of all recipients. Since home care is ideally about the melding of justice and care, and my purpose in this book is to consider how we can improve it as an ethical enterprise, it behooves us to consider the care issues that are raised by those receiving services.

### Who Receives Home Health Care?

Without exception, statistics indicate that elderly women receive the lion's share of home health services. This is primarily because women predominate over men among the elderly: According to Linda Scharer, for example, in the mid-1990s women constituted 57 percent of the age group 65–74, 63 percent of the age group 74–84, and 70 percent of the group over age 84. Unsurprisingly, this means that home care services for the elderly are largely used by women, especially since they outlive their male spouses, and as widows they are often living alone in their homes.

Of course, home health services are used by a wide variety of citizens, including disabled persons who are largely independent but require assistance with their ADLs, and young mothers who are receiving postpartum care at home. Focusing on elderly female home care recipients does not present the whole story, then, but by addressing issues for the largest, most vulnerable group with the greatest care demands, we can get at trenchant issues for the cared-for.[1]

Some of the ethical issues surrounding these elderly recipients of home health care include (1) ageist attitudes that minimize or eliminate their agency and treat them as burdens; (2) alienation from their own neighborhoods via physical and emotional isolation from their neighbors; (3) authoritarian attitudes expressed in dealings with the elderly that make it easier to take over their lives, even against their will (e.g., forcing an elderly person into a nursing home); (4) overuse or unnecessary use of technology for the aged home care recipient. This drives up the cost of their care and makes less available the attendant care hours that they urgently require; and (5) degrees of dementia that make the elderly easy targets for exploitation and theft in their homes. Given this list, and the many more ethical issues that elder home health care raises, justice requires a focus on care recipients and not just caretakers. To be sure, while caretakers deserve to be treated justly and respectfully, they may themselves be perpetrators of these wrongs, since ageism and authoritarian attitudes toward the elderly are pervasive social problems. Let us consider each of these issues in turn, then, to better understand the issues for home care recipients.

### Ageist Attitudes

Since the 1980s, and the start of an increasingly "graying" U.S. population, articles and books have focused on ageist attitudes that pervade our culture.[2] These attitudes infiltrate all aspects of society and are even applied by the elderly against themselves, who sometimes express through their own actions and attitudes vilification of aging processes.[3] Ageism is expressed in different ways, some intentional and some accidental, and results from cultural ideology. For example, chapter 1 outlines the acute care model that governs health care provision in the United States and indicates how ideologies of autonomy, independence, and self-sufficiency help guide acute care practices. Since the frail elderly fail to live up to the ideal of the "autonomous man," and since medicine cannot return them to the ideal independent self, these citizens in particular face a real paucity of care. That autonomy is the guiding principle of health care—that dependency is to be eschewed and hidden because it is embarrassing and undignified—has ageist (not to mention ableist) implications.

The focus on autonomy and independence in health care is what I consider an unintentional form of ageism; that is, it does not necessarily involve or intend discrimination against the elderly, but results in it nevertheless. Yet there are more obvious, malignant forms of ageism that do result in such discrimination, for example, names we apply to old people ("old codger," "old bag," "hag," "crone," "old biddy," "crazy old coot"). Such monikers understand aging negatively, connecting it to debilitation, decline, dementia, decrepitude, aesthetic decline, and loss. Furthermore, given the strong associations between women and the body, elderly women in particular are held up for criticism as their bodies and faces age.[4] In speaking of "loss of the admiring gaze," Sandra Bartky says:

> The loss of an admiring gaze falls disproportionately on women. We need to see but also to be seen and to be seen as attractive. Indeed, the capacity to draw admiring glances from others is a chief marker of femininity in our culture; a woman's worth, not only in the eyes of others, but in her own eyes as well, depends, to a significant degree, on her appearance. (67)

Beyond a focus on appearance, ageism serves to limit available understandings of aging and old age. Media images, popular writing, even professional writing on aging have been used to categorize, stereotype, and discipline the elderly; it serves to contain and objectify them. As Maggie Kuhn of the Gray Panthers has claimed, the biological effects of aging are not what best explain the condition of elderly people; it is rather the socioeconomic structures that serve to deprive the elderly of control over their lives, that robs them of status and power (Reinharz, 26).

Ageist attitudes toward the elderly also tend to minimize (or completely discount) their agency and treat them as burdens. For example, discussions about caretaking tend to assume that only younger women are caught in dilemmas of care for the elderly, yet elderly citizens (women especially) are increasingly carrying their own caretaking burden. Beyond spousal care, however, older women are caring in increasing numbers for their grandchildren, sometimes maintaining full guardianship of them with only meager retirement incomes for support. It is a false dichotomy, then, to separate out caretaking from care receiving, for elderly women may hold both positions at once.

Furthermore, once we get beyond our ageist assumption that the elderly are unable to reciprocate caretaking, we can begin to actually see the amount of caretaking that is being done by the elderly, specifically by women. As one commentator claims, the caretaking roles of elderly women are complicated by their own ill health, sensory loss, and financial stressors (Kayser-Jones, 136). That the elderly are both care recipients and caretakers means that we must extend justice in home care to include these caretakers-at-risk.[5]

Here Eva Kittay's notion of "doulia" is greatly valuable. Recall her argument that caretakers should be cared for within a system of nested dependencies where no caretaker is left alone and abandoned. Care for caretakers is essential where elderly caretakers are experiencing their own ill health. A system that takes advantage of women's free and low-cost caretaking is unjust. A system that exploits women's caretaking at the cost of their lives is completely immoral.

### Physical and Emotional Alienation

When considering the issues particular to elderly care recipients, we should not overlook the isolation and alienation they experience, even while living within their own communities. For a variety of reasons, including dementia, frailty, mobility problems, depression, and ageism, the elderly home care recipient is often a stranger in her own neighborhood, isolated and overlooked. In many cases I worked with clients who had no social contact whatsoever outside their interactions with me and the other home care aides. No neighbors visited, and the client could not go calling on them. In some cases, friends and neighbors would initially call on my clients (after the client returned from the hospital, for example), but after a time the neighborly visits would fall off, and clients were completely isolated again. Calling home care "community-based care" is a misnomer, then, since there is rarely any deep community participation in the elderly client's care.[6]

Elderly women especially are likely to find themselves isolated and alienated in their neighborhoods. Indeed, most of my home care clients were widowed and living alone. Their children often lived in other cities, and visits were rare. The impact of such isolation and alienation is grave, since they can lead to depression, loss of mental acuity, a loss of interest in one's surroundings, and even contemplation of suicide. My clients sorely felt their loneliness, isolation, and sense of superfluousness, especially in cases where they had defined themselves as nurturers and caretakers and were now unable to sustain these self-concepts.

Despite the isolation often experienced at home, an overwhelming proportion of the elderly population prefer it over placement in nursing homes. And there is good reason for such a preference, since despite our common conceptions, individuals in nursing homes do not always have stronger social networks and/or more social interactions. On the contrary, walking through the halls of a nursing home gives one an indication of how many residents are left alone and isolated, sitting in their wheelchairs in the hallway or watching television in bed. Since nursing homes are often understaffed, workers have little available time to exchange pleasantries with residents; as a result, residents may spend much of their time silent and alone.

Beyond this emotional alienation, elderly clients may experience physical isolation, by virtue of being shut away from the rest of their communities and by lack of physical touch. As chapter 1 indicates, home care regulations require a client to be homebound—that is, incapable of going out except for doctor's appointments—in order to receive home care services. By virtue of being mobile enough to leave her home to shop for groceries or visit neighbors, a potential client may disqualify herself from receiving the aide services she requires. One might say, then, that home care services set up the very physical isolation from which many elderly clients are suffering.

Home care recipients also lack the physical contact associated with human touch. While clients must be touched in order to be bathed and have their toiletries accomplished, this is not the kind of touching associated with caring about another. To be sure, being bathed and dressed can be pleasurable activities for clients if they are done attentively by the caretaker and not as just another task that must be completed. But often when family members are busy or distracted, and aides are on a tight time schedule, these ministrations can be more mechanical than human. So in the midst of being cared for, clients may feel a sense that they are not cared *about,* and may yearn for a pat on the hand, a back or foot rub, or an embrace. Should a well-ordered, caring society allow for such social and physical isolation? While it seems odd to claim that one has a "right" to a community, it seems less of a stretch to suggest that communities have a duty to sustain and nurture their members. Participating in community is a key aspect of human flourishing and is a need shared by all of us, even those rugged individualists who so strongly covet their independence. The old adage "out of sight, out of mind" speaks volumes. We may more easily forget the elderly simply because they are physically isolated, shut away both by restrictive home care regulations and ageist attitudes toward them. The issue of isolation indicates why we need to focus on care recipients in home care, since attending to caretakers will not directly solve the problem of social isolation.

### Authoritarian Attitudes

Authoritarian attitudes toward elderly care recipients are closely linked to the ageism mentioned earlier in this chapter. If, as I asserted, ageist assumptions, stereotypes, and ideologies undergird much of our thinking about the elderly—including stereotypes that suggest the elderly are mentally infirm—then it is not a large step from there to treating the elderly in dismissive and authoritarian ways.

What is really wrong with authoritarian attitudes toward the elderly, especially when in some cases such authoritarianism may be called for? These attitudes deny persons their own perspectives on what is good for them. Barring cases where individuals are completely incompetent and are no longer capable of effectively making self-regarding decisions, we all have a basic interest in directing our lives. By treating persons in authoritarian ways we deny their full status as members of the moral community. And, from a feminist perspective, treating elderly women in an authoritarian manner represents an extension of patriarchal thinking, since women's self-regarding choices are already denied and overlooked in masculinist culture.[7] Feminists have been concerned about both our culture's overemphasis on autonomy (especially in health care ethics) and the denial of women's attempts at autonomy. They have argued that autonomy is "king of the hill" in bioethics and should be weighed against other important values like relationships, justice, and beneficence; at the same time, they have argued for respecting women's autonomy in a culture that all too readily dismisses their attempts to govern their own lives. In the case of elderly female home care recipients, we should note these feminist concerns and take special care to respect the choices of these vulnerable citizens.

Elderly persons are acquainted with and terrified of authoritarian treatment. Indeed, in some cases it takes on legendary proportions. For example, one home care client with whom I worked related a story about a woman in her apartment complex who was told by her son that they would take a day trip together to check out a nursing home; the client told me "she never came back." Her son had secretly packed her bag and without her knowledge had set up her permanent residency in the nursing home. Whether or not the events really unfolded in this way, the conspiratorial manner in which the woman relayed this story spoke volumes about her own worries that such a thing could happen to her. Authoritarian attitudes are widespread enough that the elderly have good reason to be concerned.

It is often easy to take authoritarian attitudes to the elderly, especially if they are female, frail, demented, frightened, or depressed. In fact, as I suggested above, there are times when such an attitude may be necessary: when a client refuses to bathe for days on end, for example. In one case, I worked with a demented client who refused to bathe at all. When aides tried to get her out of bed to have a shower, she would scream, bite, and spit at them. This client's bodily odor became so strong that it was repugnant to sit with her to read or talk. There was also a concern about infection, since she was bedridden and not getting proper genital care. I found the only way to accomplish her bath (which was one of the very purposes for which I was sent to her home) was to take an authoritarian approach, since reasoning and pleading with Mrs. Gilroy did not work. Similarly, when sent to a hospital to help feed an 85-year-old Asian man whose weight was dropping, I found it necessary to pop the spoon in his mouth against his obvious protestations. (Although he did not speak English, he made it clear that he did not appreciate my ministrations!) There were times that I felt uncomfortable with the authoritarian approach, but in some cases it was necessary for the clients' good, as well as those working with them.[8]

We need to take care, then, in determining when authoritarian attitudes are justified and when they are not. It is not always clear how to determine the distinction. For instance, I am still uncertain as to whether my force-feeding of the elderly Asian client was appropriate. Perhaps he was worn out, eating was exhausting, and his refusal to eat was perfectly reasonable. His family and the nurses on the ward certainly did not think so. Indeed, it was the family who paid for an aide's services at meal times, since the nurses were too busy to feed him. But since he wanted to return home, and the hospital would not release him until he gained some weight, my actions seemed justified so that he would reach his goal of being discharged.

I do not think there is a formula for determining when authoritarian attitudes toward the elderly care recipient are justified and when they are not. Generally, where clients refuse nursing home care and demand to stay in their own homes, we have an obligation to cooperate because so much is at stake for that client. Choosing the place and manner in which one lives, and the kinds of relationships one wishes to engage in, are some of the most important choices one can make, and they seriously impact one's life enjoyment. However, this obligation is not absolute, since the client may be too confused, frail, or ill to remain at home. Furthermore, the request to remain at home must be balanced against the interests of the client's neighbors, who may also be put at risk if she forgets to turn off burners or irons or fails to extinguish cigarettes. At the very least, we should enable the client to remain at home for as long as possible, taking measures that will extend her ability to remain there.

In her work on home care, Nancy Dubler distinguishes between autonomy and accommodation, asserting the importance of accommodation to the home care context.

> In the context of home care it makes far more sense to talk not about *autonomy* but about *accommodation,* about mediating the patient's desires by the reality of the available services and the real and weighty competing interests of others. (159)

We need, then, to accommodate the expressed wishes of clients insofar as they are capable and competent to make self-regarding claims.[9] But this is not a black-or-white issue: Competency comes in degrees, and clients may be competent in some areas of their lives but not in others. I will say more about this in chapter 5, where I will consider how to negotiate relationships within home health care.

### Overusing Medical Technology in Home Health Care

Another ethical issue that a detailed account of elder home care should treat is the use of medical technology in the home setting. Recall that home health care was initially instituted as a cost-saving measure. Because long hospital stays are expensive, and the costs of medical technology are driving up the cost of hospital care, the move to home care was seen as a way of avoiding the high costs. Some supporters of home care have touted it as a cheaper, better alternative. As I have argued, it is cheaper because of the exploitation of women caretakers. But home care was also initially cheaper because the same high-tech interventions were not applied to patients in the home as they were in the hospital. However, this is changing, and increasingly the client's home is becoming more institutional as more medical technology is invoked. As William Ruddick has queried, "Miniaturized or simplified ventilators, drug and nutrition-infusion devices, various monitors, and other hospital equipment are making this shift from hospital to home feasible, even for seriously dependent patients. How desirable is this shift?" (166).

I resist the move toward high-tech home health care, as it raises the cost such that many clients who need care cannot afford it. Such technological measures also change the moral landscape for home care, making it increasingly institutional and less like home, thus thwarting its very purpose. As Lidia Pousada claims, high-tech home care changes what it means to give quality care, because quality of care is reduced to the power and accuracy of machines (107). Since high-tech home care changes the quality of the home, one must wonder where one finds the "home" in high-tech home care.

First, I will consider the kinds of high-tech home care that are currently in use, and then I will indicate why I consider many of them problematic. I should emphasize that my concern is less with *rationing* scarce medical resources than with how best to meet the home care needs of care recipients. I contend that high-tech approaches will generally fail in this regard, since elderly clients identify their care needs in terms of caretaking rather than cutting-edge technology.

Technology has been applied in the home care setting to enable an increasing number of patients to complete medical care at home. Several technologies have become prevalent in the care of elderly persons, including decubitus care with air-fluidized beds, catheterization of the urinary tract, total parenteral nutrition and enteral feeding tubes, intravenous antibiotics, home infusion pumps for patient-controlled analgesia, chronic ambulatory peritoneal dialysis, and home respirators and/or home oxygen therapy. While use of these technologies raises pressing bioethical questions regarding the maintenance of quality of life versus artificial extension of life, I here intend to consider them in relation to the goals of home health care. I contend that while some of these technologies may be justified because they are minimally invasive, relatively simple, and improve the quality of clients' lives such that they can better engage with their loved ones and communities, others should not be used because they are highly invasive (both for the client's body and for normal functioning within the home) and extremely complex.

Consider, for example, decubitus at-home care. Pressure sores are a recurring problem for geriatric home care clients and are correlated with chronic debilitating disease. "There is a sixfold increase in mortality when a pressure sore develops in an older patient; it is not clear whether this is because the development of pressure sores correlates with the presence of severe multisystemic disease or because pressure sores themselves cause an increase in mortality" (Pousada, 111). Treatment of these ulcers in the home setting requires large resource commitments via personnel and medication/equipment. Like home health care spending, most of the costs for decubitus care are borne by Medicare, since it is the growing elderly population that experiences the most serious problems with pressure sores. And increasingly, the way that decubitus care is carried out is through use of high-tech beds that were once limited to the hospital setting. Through the use of alternating-pressure air mattresses and air-fluidized beds, pressure on damaged tissues is reduced so that healing can occur. Such beds also eliminate the friction caused by lying on traditional mattresses, reduce bacterial growth and pain, and better ensure the comfort of clients. These beds significantly reduce decubitus ulcers in the elderly. Yet high-tech beds are an example of the heavy artillery available through home care services. Such beds rent for $50 to $200 per day, and they have a purchase price of between $20,000 and $35,000. As Pousada claims, "The use of these beds in the home care setting appears to result in a decrease in rehospitalizations and a greater capacity to adhere to DRG limits, which translates into some savings for hospitals but not for Medicare" (112).

Air-fluidized beds and alternating-pressure air mattresses have been used to great effect on burn victims and patients with post-acute injuries. The efficacy of these beds for the advanced elderly who are often immobilized, debilitated, or suffering dementia is questionable, however. When used at great cost on clients with poor long-term prognoses, such technology appears less justified.[10] Furthermore, in the turn to such heavy medical artillery, "their cost, size, weight, and maintenance costs have caused them to be dubbed the 'BMWs of decubitus care'" (Pousada, 113).

Catheterization of the urinary tract is another technology that is currently in use in the home care setting. For a variety of reasons, the elderly develop urinary problems. These are addressed by urinary tract catheterization, which maintains the normal flow of urine. Such catheterization is inexpensive, and family members and medical personnel can easily learn to insert and empty them. While some medical oversight is required, this technology is simple enough and minimally invasive such that it can greatly improve the quality of the client's home life.

High-tech home health care is also marked by the use of nasogastric feeding tubes, percutaneous enteral gastrostomy (PEG) tubes, or home parenteral nutrition (HPN) to ensure proper nutritional support. Following strokes or the onset of dementia, elderly clients have a much more difficult time meeting their nutritional needs; in such cases, they may require a special feeding, since intake by mouth may be impossible. While nasogastic and PEG tubes are quite effective and relatively inexpensive, HPN is an extremely expensive option ($75,000 to $150,000 per patient per year). We must question under what circumstances HPN should be offered and what our goals are in providing such care.

By considering different forms of high-tech home care, we get a sense of the wide spectrum of technology. While some forms may be justified (urinary tract catheterization, for example), others may not because they are extremely costly, invasive, and destructive of the home environment. Furthermore, these measures relate back to the dominant medical paradigm of control and cure that governs medicine at the macro level. Yet despite this paradigm, what many elderly home care clients want most is the assistance and comfort of another human being, not complicated equipment and medications that must be heavily monitored and that require special training.

As I argued in chapter 2, we need to be clear about the goals of home health care. If it is intended to be nothing more than a different place for offering the same high-tech, institutional-style care, then incorporating cutting-edge technology into home care practice may be justified. If it is to be differentiated from the technologically based acute care found in hospitals, however, then we may want to reconsider the coming of expensive technology to home health care. I argue that a philosophy best suited to the home care setting is one that treats patients as whole beings with a past, present, and future. High-tech interventions may interfere with this understanding of home care by focusing our attention on the technology rather than the person to whom the technology is connected. It has the potential to turn the home into an alien, frightening place that the client connects with pain and suffering rather than comfort and intimacy.[11]

### Degrees of Dementia

Many elderly home care clients suffer dementia, which renders them particularly vulnerable to the actions and choices of others. This is perhaps one of the most pressing problems in home care, as it raises a host of issues involving power and domination. For example, cases often arise where clients are swindled by aides because the aides are able to gain access to the clients' bank accounts and private monies. Or in some cases of familial care, clients may be put at risk by family members yet be too afraid or befuddled to report the risky behaviors. In both cases, clients are subjected to great harm, both economic and personal, and home care appears to be a dangerous enterprise. While abuse and exploitation of patients with dementia may occur in institutional settings, it is far less likely, since a variety of people are in contact with them. There is at least some monitoring of patients in nursing homes given the public nature of nursing home care. In the home care setting, however, where few people are in contact with or have access to clients, it is far easier to get away with unethical behavior that can do serious harm.

The exploitation of demented elderly home care clients arose in my home care practice. In one case, a neighbor who had been helping my client by cutting grass and doing small repairs was caught stealing items from the client's home. He had keys to her house and would come and go as he pleased, over time removing a number of valuable antiques. The client, who was very confused, did not know that this was going on; furthermore, she insisted on continuing private visits with her neighbor, even though he would steal money from her, sometimes taking money out of her jewelry box, sometimes having her write checks for him. Eventually the home care office stopped the private interviews, and he was refused entry to the client's home. But this only occurred after the neighbor had seriously abused the client's trust and taken advantage of her vulnerability.

Such violations also occur at the hands of home care workers. Given the high turnover rate in the home care workforce and the scarcity of new recruits, some studies indicate that workers with criminal records can end up as unlicensed aides in clients' homes. For example, as one report claims, an underground network exists by which families can hire home care aides for much lower pay than the standard industry cost. But such aides are uncertified, untrained, and have not undergone a criminal background check. There is no way of regulating such workers (Layton and Zambito).

Thus, both caretakers and care recipients are harmed by the kind of home care system currently in place. Under our system, the most positive aspect—the caretaker/client relationship—is perverted by poverty-level wages and a resulting revolving door workforce that place clients and paid caretakers at odds with one another. It is unsurprising that some aides are willing to take advantage of their clients, since they, too, are abused and exploited by the home care system.

All the issues I have outlined come together to raise questions about care and justice. Clearly, home health care requires caring for and about vulnerable citizens, including both caretakers and care recipients. A system that encourages people to care for mercenary reasons is going to fail as much as a system that encourages altruistic caring. While I am critical of ideologies that render women responsible for caretaking and that encourage dangerous forms of self-abnegation, I also reject a system of home care founded on an overemphasis on justice. For example, while social support

for caretakers requires livable wages and benefits for them, this does not ex-
haust questions of caring. If caretakers provide care only because of the pay,
then the focus may become caring for clients: Caring *about* them may fall
by the wayside. And as I argued in chapter 2, home health care amounts to
much more than handling bodies and cleaning homes for money. Indeed,
the work of a home care aide is as much a calling as primary school teaching or entering the priesthood. Practitioners ought to enter these professions
not for monetary reasons but because they feel called to do so. Nel Noddings distinguishes between what she calls "ethical caring," or "caring that
has to be summoned—by obedience to duty and principle in Kantian ethics,
by reminders of an ideal self in caring," and "natural caring," or "caring
out of love or inclination." She claims that ethical caring comes out of natural caring and that the purpose of ethical caring is to restore natural care.
Furthermore, Noddings argues, to offer the most humane, nurturing care in
home care we ought to be focusing on natural caring, since ethical caring
can be cold and impersonal, and "astute recipients of care can often detect
a subtle difference" (1995, 151–52).

### *Balancing Interests: Understanding Selves as Relational*

While it may sometimes seem like the interests of the caretaker
(both paid and familial) and those of the cared-for are in conflict, I argue
that this only appears to be the case. To be sure, clients and caretakers come
into conflict in the home as they attempt to negotiate the mundane activities of daily life and as they each try to maintain some semblance of control
in a home care system that robs them of it. But I reject the notion that caretakers and care recipients have clashing interests at any deep level or that
they must struggle against one another for ascendancy. Rather, taking a relational approach to autonomy, I see the interests of caretakers and cared-
for as enmeshed. By improving working conditions for home care aides and
providing social support for family caretakers, we improve conditions for
the client. And as we take steps to ensure the comfort and safety for clients
in their homes, we improve conditions for those in relationship to the care
recipient. To take a simple example, if a client's home is impoverished such
that no buckets, mops, and cleaning supplies are available, then I, as the
aide, will not be able to provide the kind of clean living conditions I would
desire for her. But if a state agency ensures that the elderly client has a home
well stocked with nutritious food and cleaning supplies, then I am positioned to do my job well. Similarly, if as an aide I am poorly remunerated
for my work, lacking health insurance and sick leave, then my tenure in the
home care profession is likely to be brief and my clients will have much

more difficulty securing caretakers as I (and other workers) move in and out of the industry.

By rejecting the conflictual model of the client/aide relationship, we can consider a more symbiotic approach that does not understand relationships as problems to be solved. But to do this we need a better understanding of what a relational account of autonomy looks like and how such an understanding can better identify the importance of both autonomy and human relationships. To this end, I will consider some recent feminist accounts of relational autonomy, ones that understand us as primarily beings-in-relationship. These accounts follow and expand upon the care ethics I outlined in chapter 3.

As Linda Barclay claims,

> Numerous moral and political theories promote a vision of the autonomous self as essentially independent and self-sufficient, a vision that denies the inescapable connectedness of selves and the fact that their immersion in networks of relationships forms their desires, aspirations, indeed their very identities. In other words, what is denied is that the self is essentially social. (52)

As Barclay and other feminists argue, the self *is* essentially social, meaning that who I am, my identity, is derived from socialization processes and the relationships into which I am born. As Annette Baier phrases it, we are all "second persons," skilled in the art of personhood through relationships of dependency that we share with others. She indicates that each individual's life history—and our collective human history—depends upon each of us having a childhood where a cultural heritage is transmitted (84–85). Thus, we do not become autonomous persons despite our relationships with others but because of them. And as Eva Kittay has indicated, liberal theories that understand selves as primarily independent and self-sufficient do violence to the relational quality of our selves and our autonomy.

A relational conception of autonomy is well suited to the enterprise of home health care. Instead of understanding selves as "islands unto themselves," and processes of individuation as setting us apart from one another, relational autonomy sees our selves as developing out of the relationships in which we are enmeshed. While a relational conception of autonomy does not deny that autonomy is possible—it resists situating the self as wholly social such that no authentic self-regarding choices are possible—it sees autonomy as developing out of relationship. This is certainly reflected in the home care setting, where clients' selves are intimately tied to the quality of relationships with their family caretakers and home care workers. A relational approach to autonomy works best in home care because it can be applied to both familial caretaking relationships and formal care relationships.

Relational autonomy matters here because, as James and Hilde Lindemann Nelson claim, *families* matter. It is by being part of families that we become fully flourishing selves (or, in cases of bad family situations, we become stunted, underdeveloped selves). As the Nelsons assert,

> When we live in close and affectionate proximity with others, we can be seen and celebrated specially; we can be known more fully than our relationships in the workplace, in civic life, or in casual friendships permit. Being known well—being seen lovingly and particularly, in a way that singles us out from the billions of others who walk in the world—reinforces our understanding of who we are. As our intimates respond to what they come to know of us, we turn their response into a fuller knowledge of ourselves. By the same token, if we are not seen lovingly, we learn to accept whatever negative image of ourselves our family happens to offer; especially when we are children, but also when we are grown, those with whom we live in intimacy have a terrible power over us. (37)

This power can be used for good or ill, can lead to human flourishing or devastation, but in either case must be accounted for in home care. Many clients are living with their extended families where interests are entangled such that asserting client autonomy fails to capture the relational aspect of it. Families not only form in our early years the kinds of selves that we become; they offer a means of maintaining identities as adults, too.

For example, during times of illness, families can serve to keep our selves together. When illness leaves us at sea because we are out of synch with our normal existence, they can provide the grounding we need to keep us tied to our identities.[12] During periods of transition, families provide the narratives and histories that give content to who we are and that allow us to put our selves back together. Susan Brison has written on trauma and the ways in which relationships serve to reconstruct selves following a traumatic event. Referring to her own recovery from trauma, Brison writes that selves are "remade" by caring for others and being cared for. Relationships sustain and often reconstruct our sense of self.

These authors raise another aspect of relationships and families that sustain us: They provide us with narratives (sometimes even new ones) that make us who we are. People relate narratives all the time. A classic example is the forgetful elderly person who tells the same stories over and over again. While this can be frustrating and tedious for those who hear the narratives repeatedly, it indicates the power of stories in situating us as whole persons. In institutional settings, we often get only "time slices" of patients such that they are not particular persons with rich histories; institutional caretakers are not often introduced to the details of patients' lives. Narratives become essential to patients at such times, as they signal to others that they have a past, that they mean something to particular others, and that they are worth caring about.

In the home care setting, however, one usually gets a better sense of the client's history because everywhere one finds reminders of the *person*. The objects within clients' homes (their family photographs, trinkets, musical instruments, magazines, antiques, and so on) tell us much about the client as a person, and at times family members themselves will fill in the gaps. Beyond these physical reminders, clients relate narratives during the many hours aides spend with them, giving a context for their lives: "I was a school teacher in 1923"; or "My husband and I traveled to Europe for our honeymoon in 1934 when I was 18 years old"; or "My daughter, Sylvia, has always been so distant. I wish she would call more often." These narratives can be crucial to the effective provision of home care, as they humanize and particularize clients in ways that make them real persons to the workers and not just bodies that require attention.

So while home care workers are not involved in the early formation of clients' selves, they are nevertheless an important part of the maintenance of selves. Like familial caretakers, their relationships with clients can also be understood from a model of relational autonomy. As what can reasonably be termed "intimates" with their clients, aides have the power through their words and actions to either support or destroy their clients' selves. Aides see and hear things that reveal much about the client, and these bits of information are sometimes crucial to understanding and accommodating them. Indeed, as I indicated in chapter 2, some home care theorists have applied a familial ethic to the client/aide relationship, given the alacrity with and degree to which aides become viewed as part of the client's family. For example, when interviewed, one home care aide claimed, "'My client has become like my mother'" (Chichin, 173).

That home care workers are treated as fictive kin, and that they may feel deep connections to their clients, highlights that home care's virtues are also its vices. As many studies show, it is these kinds of connections that makes home care fulfilling and satisfying work. But such relationships also make workers vulnerable to the inadvertent exploitation by clients, who are allotted so few hours of formal care. As Eileen Chichin's study shows, a large proportion of home care workers put in extra hours without pay, usually for relational reasons (172–73). As I argued in chapter 3, the altruism already associated with "women's work" complicates women's experiences as formal caretakers. Add to this the kinds of personal attachments formed through home care relationships, and one can see how aides become deeply committed to their clients. As Karner puts it, with status as honorary family members come obligations. Aides may take on obligations that go well beyond a contractual model of human relationships. One "contracts" to take care of a client in her home for a certain number of hours; one does not "contract" to bring cookies, stay beyond paid hours, attend the clients' family gatherings, or care about the client as a whole person.

Though the term *client* may suggest a highly contractual home care relationship, the client/aide relationship cannot be captured by such a model. This is why a concept of relational autonomy is useful here, for it best characterizes the nature of many client/aide relationships. While not all such pairings are harmonious (since some clients and paid caretakers have damaging relationships), many are. This means that even paid caretakers understand who they are as deeply connected to the clients they serve. Note, for example, the way in which my own self-understandings are connected to relationships I had with clients. I still define who I am, the kind of person I am becoming, and who I want to be in connection with clients who played a serious role in my development. I hope it is obvious through the narratives I relate in this book that over time my clients' stories became *my* stories; the narratives I relate herein served to define a certain period of my life and helped determine the kind of philosopher I became. It is erroneous, then, to compartmentalize our lives. My work self was not separable from my scholarly/educated self, as the issues I witnessed in my work life directly impacted the focus of my professional work.

Likewise, other home care aides cannot easily separate their work as aides from their personal lives. On the contrary, the work becomes personal as relationships with clients develop. A beloved client who is ailing can keep an aide awake at night worrying; and in a similar fashion, clients may feel the weight of their aides' personal problems, worrying about them long after the aides' shifts are over. While such relationships of natural caring are really what home care ought to be about, we must also guard against deep bonds being used as an excuse for poorly paying caretakers (as formal caretakers) or for not remunerating them at all (as family caretakers). In addition, such bonds should not result in ill, demented, or emotionally strained clients becoming financially or personally involved in aides' lives.

Just because caretaker/client relationships are formed in the home setting does not mean they lack a social and political aspect. Home care straddles the privacy of the home and the public realm such that even familial home care arrangements raise public concerns; thus, home care points out the myth of the public/private split. For example, the move toward paid family caretaking raises important political issues concerning the provision of quality care for elderly citizens: What should we do when paid family caretakers (who are essentially "employees" for their loved ones) are failing to provide decent quality care? It is to such questions that I will turn in chapter 5.

Since home care relationships are neither simply contractual nor personal relationships, we need a more nuanced understanding of them. Aides and clients both must have exit options for getting out of uncomfortable or destructive home care relationships. If a client becomes uncomfortable with her home care aide because the aide crosses boundaries, or if an aide finds a caretaking relationship too intense or demanding to sustain, then measures must be in place to allow parties to defuse or exit the relationship. This is not to revert to a contractual way of thinking where the two parties contract for mutual benefit; it is only to recognize the complexity of home-based care, where client and aide are more than just contracting parties but less than family. This is why a public or politicized care ethic should guide our thinking: We need enough justice within such relationships to protect and sustain the bonds of care that are created through the practice of home health care.

If we take seriously a relational autonomy approach, we can more effectively address issues for care recipients. This melds with the concept of accommodation that Nancy Dubler recommends for home care: taking clients' requests seriously, and being obliged to respond, but placing those requests in a relational context. While I think such a notion of accommodation is useful beyond the home care setting, it is especially important in that arena, where interests are deeply connected and bald autonomy claims may be problematic and damaging to others.

### Conclusion

Chapters 3 and 4 offer frameworks that can act as foundations for ethics in home health care. These chapters indicate the need for (1) tempering care with justice in home care, allowing for the flourishing of meaningful client/caretaker relationships, and (2) understanding autonomy as relational rather than the choices arrived at independently by a lone agent. By applying these frameworks, I am arguing, we can consider important issues like the exploitation of caretakers based on a perversion of the care ethic, the authoritarian attitudes that are taken with care recipients, and even broader questions like the kind of home health care system we want to support.

But these frameworks do not explicitly direct us regarding what to do when difficult ethical issues arise in the home care setting—for example, how aides should respond when loving clients want to give them money and other gifts; what to do when clients refuse to take medications at home or follow medical advice; how to negotiate situations where paid family caretakers are not doing their job; how to react to clients' family members who interfere with the aides' caretaking; and when (and if) paid caretakers should enter dangerous workplaces (like gang-dominated neighborhoods) to do their jobs. I do think that these two frameworks offer a moral compass for negotiating ethical dilemmas, and in the following chapter I will consider a variety of such dilemmas, some quite mundane, that challenge ethicists and practitioners in home health care.

# 5 The Personal Is Political

*Negotiating Relationships within the Home Care Setting*

As I argued in chapter 4, a feminist conception of relational autonomy best characterizes the home care relationships between clients, families, and paid caretakers. But such a conception of autonomy also impacts the moral judgments we make about home care. If human beings are, as feminists claim, interdependent beings, and if our very identities come out of the relationships in which we are involved, then we ought to judge home care by the quality of the relationships in question and the way in which the choices we make with, for, and about people will affect their identities. So, for example, in attempting to make a moral judgment about whether to remove an elderly home care client from her beloved home, we must consider such an action in terms of the impact on that woman's self-understandings and her relationships with others. A relational conception of autonomy leads us to consider not just practical moral questions about client safety and efficient caretaking but also the impact of our actions on identities and relationships.

I have largely based my critique of home care on a feminist theory that is critical of the public/private split. I have also offered a feminist theory of the state that argues for a change in the way that we understand the relationship between the state and its female citizens. But one might still wonder how feminist ethics addresses the daily personal issues that arise within the home care setting. It is one thing to claim that feminist ethics can lead us to different conclusions about the morality of home health care on a macrolevel; it is another thing to claim that it differently addresses personal conflicts and tensions that may arise in home care situations.

A feminist approach provides a different lens from which to judge the morality of home care relationships. Rather than a universalistic, principled approach to such relationships, I advocate a contextualized, concrete one. What this means is that one cannot judge the quality of these intimate relationships based on an objective understanding of acceptable behaviors within the home care industry. Once real people are taken into consideration, moral judgments become rich and complex. It may not be so clear whether the right thing to do is to take an elderly woman out of her home (even though in a supervisor's best judgment, that woman is not getting the best care) if the woman does not want to leave it. This chapter will deal with a variety of such relational considerations that arise in the home care setting and offer some direction as to what we should do about them.

The received view of autonomy and the autonomous self fail to adequately represent real selves in the real world. The relational approach to autonomy taken by many feminists, conversely, treats us as selves-in-relationships, where these relationships are largely constitutive of the selves that we become. This feminist conception of autonomy also takes seriously the extent to which social institutions, social values, and gender role socialization affect the choices and actions of the autonomous agent.

There are almost endless relational moral issues that arise in the home care setting; this book couldn't possibly account for all of them. In what follows, then, I will take a sampling of issues that either arose in my own practice, that were related to me by other aides, or that are raised as serious concerns in the literature on home care. The problems I address range from the mundane to the most pressing, but they all share one thing in common: They come out of the intimate relationships that are formed within the home care setting.

### Gift Giving and the Question of Reciprocity

Issues about gift giving—the ethics of accepting gifts from clients—arose in my own home care experiences and are common problems. On several occasions, clients offered me gifts to show their gratitude. The offerings ranged from money to tiny crystal figurines, books, and food. In one situation, a client with whom I became very friendly offered on my very last shift an envelope with a card inside. I opened it in front of him to find a check for $100 enclosed. My home care agency had strict rules about accepting gifts: One was simply not allowed to do so. Knowing this, and feeling awkward, I held the check out and mumbled that I couldn't accept his gift, though I was very grateful. The client seemed disappointed but retrieved the check. When I returned home, my mother severely admonished me for refusing the man's gift; as she put it, it was "like throwing it back in his face."

In another case, an elderly client with fairly severe dementia began offering me gifts upon each visit I made to her home. She had a glass display case with beautiful little crystal figurines inside, and with each shift she would put one in my hand, telling me to take it home. Each time she did this, after I helped her to bed, I would replace the figurine in the glass case. We played out this scenario over and over again; she never seemed to notice that I never accepted her offerings.

In yet another situation, the sister of a client—again, someone with whom I'd formed a close bond—bestowed upon me a beautiful book on house plants with a thank-you card tucked inside. This woman knew that I loved plants, and we had often discussed my lack of a green thumb. As a final thanks for my help, she gave me the book; it was clear to me that she had gone out of her way to find something that would be meaningful to me.

How is one to determine the morality of accepting gifts in such cases? One could take the principled approach held by my employer that one is never to accept gifts from clients. Such an approach certainly protects against charges of theft, fraud, abuse of clients, and so forth. But notice the other effect of such an approach: It denies clients the right to participate in an important aspect of relationship, namely, reciprocity. In the three cases above, I can report that I am still conflicted about rejecting the client's check; I am confident in the moral appropriateness of rejecting my demented client's offering of crystal figurines; and I am certain that I did the right thing in accepting the book from my client's sister. Is there any universal principle that I am applying in making these determinations? The answer is no.

The judgments I have formed about the moral rightness or wrongness of my actions is not based on any universal principle (like "never accept money, but objects are acceptable" or "don't ever take gifts from people who lack full mental capacity"). Rather, they are based on my sense of the relationships, the possibility of reciprocity in each case, and the likely outcomes of accepting the gift.

My client with dementia, for example, did not have presence of mind to be capable of engaging in reciprocity as we commonly understand it. So I understood her constant offerings as inauthentic because she wasn't capable of forming the intentions that undergird gift giving. Indeed, her adult children informed me that they had been forced to seek power of attorney over her finances, as the woman had been writing checks to numerous charities, sometimes leaving nothing behind for her rent, groceries, or utilities. When pressed for a rationale, my client could not remember having written the checks to the charities. Under such circumstances, it is morally questionable for one to accept another's offerings, since the gift is not based on an authentic desire for reciprocity and it is possible, and even likely, that the individual may later panic because she was "robbed."

In my acceptance of the book, however, no such concerns were present. The woman who offered it had deliberately and thoughtfully purchased the book for me. It was an attempt to give something back and to recognize the work that I had done for her and her ailing sister. To refuse to accept the book would have been insulting and immoral; the rejection would symbolize a refusal of reciprocity or (to put it another way) my desire to maintain a strictly one-sided, formal relationship.

I remain conflicted about the offering of money because I do worry that, as my mother put it, my refusal was equivalent to throwing the gift back in my client's face or rejecting reciprocity. This male client was reciprocating in perhaps the only way he knew how—or the only way in which he was capable. He did not bake, crochet, or go shopping, so his ability to offer me something of a nonmonetary nature was limited. And since the offering was done in the spirit of relationship, not out of a tit-for-tat sensibility, my refusal to take the money was more than just the falling-through of a financial transaction. It symbolized my rejection of reciprocity.

Feminist theorists have written on the nature of reciprocity and the importance of *receiving* as well as giving. For example, Nel Noddings indicates that receiving is an ethical act, and like other ethical requirements, one can fail miserably to fulfill it. As she states,

> This attitude of warm acceptance and trust is important to all caring relationships. . . . When this attitude is missed, the one who is the object of caretaking feels like an object. He is being treated, handled by formula. . . . To be treated as "types" instead of individuals, to have strategies exercised on us, objectifies us. We become "cases" instead of persons. (1996, 27)

To have ethical caring, and an ethical basis for home care policies like gift giving, we must be responsive to this question of reciprocity. Nothing is more humiliating and psychically harmful than to have one's attempts at reciprocity summarily rejected. For example, a client's refusal to accept my care sometimes stung more than the occasional slaps I received from clients with dementia. This is because, in order to be completed, my act of caring had to be taken up by others.

But in the home care arena, the caretaker gives in ways that are tangible, recognizable, and beneficial. The same cannot always be true of the cared-for. In some cases, the cared-for suffer dementia, Alzheimer's disease, or severe mental disabilities, and they are not capable of recognizing or returning care.[1] In other situations, they are too ill to show thanks. And in still others, clients are often too poor to have much to offer. In recognizing this imbalance in ability to give, one becomes sensitized to the meaningfulness of clients' attempts to give back, in sometimes simple ways. The offering of a plate of cookies, for example, takes on far more meaning, and so, by extension, does the refusal to accept them.

As I have been arguing, it is difficult to make a principled case against gift giving in the home care setting. For once we take seriously the moral concerns for responsiveness and reciprocity, we begin to see the moral damage that can be done by refusing to accept clients' offerings. As Marilyn Friedman has argued, it may be *immoral* to allow principled commitments to always determine our interactions with those with whom we are in relationships of care.

I think Friedman is right that we should not subject people we care about (or care for) to scrutiny according to abstract standards. However, one might wonder how we are then to adjudicate between morally good forms of gift giving and reciprocity and morally bad ones. Recall the client I mentioned in chapter 4 who was being systematically robbed by her neighbor, someone she considered a friend. This woman, Mrs. G, was confused, suffering the early stages of Alzheimer's disease, and quite vulnerable. So while she would freely give cash and sometimes checks to her neighbor, such "gift giving" was taking place within a negative context of care. The neighbor's engagement with Mrs. G was not based on a caring, nurturing relationship of reciprocity (however unequal the parties' capacities to reciprocate may have been). His whole purpose was to defraud Mrs. G of as much of her property and money as he could before the home care agency discovered his activities. The contextual features of such exploitation differ so vastly from the cases I previously mentioned that it is hard to imagine a moral agent could not make the distinction between "good" and "bad" gift giving and receiving.

As Friedman points out, not every relationship contributes to integrity and fulfillment:

> Personal relationships vary widely in their moral value. The quality of a particular relationship is profoundly important in determining the moral

worth of any partiality which is necessary for sustaining that relationship. To the extent that partiality is a duty in close personal relationships, it is a prima facie duty only, to be fully assessed, among other things, in light of the moral worth of the particular relationships it helps to preserve. (40)

Thus, by arguing from a contextualist basis for the ethics of gift giving, I am not simply abandoning vulnerable clients to potential fraud and abuse. Not any and all cases of gift giving are morally supportable, and while I am not willing to morally condemn even offers of monetary gifts, I think we must understand the likely effects of such offerings. Taking a $100 bonus from a wealthy client who clearly expresses her desire to reciprocate your care is different in kind than accepting $100 from a moderately to severely demented client who is barely able to subsist on her monthly pension. The lesson in considering this issue is that, though "lowly" workers, home care aides are moral agents who should be empowered to make contextual determinations regarding the morality of accepting gifts. Such determinations should not be done in secret or private, however, but should be done through discourse with other aides, the home care office, and, ideally, clients themselves.

The moral considerations surrounding gift giving in home care relate to the serious problem of racism that sometimes surfaces at the level of care provision. Once again, concerns arise about relationship and identity and about the deep connections between reciprocity and positive self-concepts. It is to the moral issue of racism in home care to which I will now turn.

### The Problem of Racist Clients

As chapter 1 indicates, the home care industry in the United States is dominated at the entry level by minority female workers. This fact raises acute relational problems when clients and prospective clients refuse care from women of color. And it is not uncommon for clients to make such refusals, especially in their own homes, where they may experience "emboldened autonomy"[2] and they are arguably free to express their own prejudices and stereotypes. Again, those involved in home care uniquely experience the tension created by the clashing of the "private" sphere of home with the "public" sphere of work and politics.

There has not been common agreement on what is the correct moral response to racist attitudes and demands. Some theorists argue that white clients who request (or demand) a worker of the same race should not be accommodated and should have their preference emphatically and soundly rejected. Others argue that, given the home setting, individuals should be free to make judgments regarding who will enter their homes and under what circumstances. Again, while I do not offer any principled moral response to racist clients, I do think that a feminist moral approach offers some important guideposts for thinking through such requests.

First, one must ask whether individuals should be free to be bigots. This is a controversial question, especially in light of the history of racism and outright hatred that has targeted African Americans. Indeed, in our current legal and political climate, we have encoded laws to protect African Americans and women against discrimination. These laws apply to the public realm of work and politics: One is not entitled to bar a woman or black from a job by virtue of her gender or race; one cannot bar African Americans from public services; and women and blacks are now extended equal rights to education.

These laws do not apply, however, within the four walls of individual homes. There, people are free to express discriminatory or idiosyncratic preferences regarding who comes into their homes and for what purposes. Taken in concert with the problem of client and caretaker powerlessness in a largely impersonal system and the intimate and personal nature of the tasks being accomplished, ethicist Adrienne Asch argues that a client's request for a certain kind of worker should be taken seriously. She says:

> If the client believes she cannot be comfortable with a suggested person based on anything—personality or appearance, speaking style, ethnicity, or race—those wishes must be honored. It makes no sense to insist that a talkative client work with someone who wants little social interaction if a more communicative worker can be found. Similarly, it makes no sense to insist that black clients work with white assistants (or vice versa) if they have strong reservations about doing so and if other people are available. Case managers and agencies are understandably wary of honoring their clients' racial and ethnic preferences. Individuals have not been lynched or enslaved for being talkative as they have been for being black, and thus, the types of preferences are not absolutely identical. Our legacy of racism continues to deny people meaningful life. Yet the particular client who needs help must not bear all the consequences of this history at the price of her own well-being. . . . In their own homes, even people who need help must be free to be bigots. (229)

Asch's argument is not based on a minimal conception of negative rights, where individuals are free to make choices without interference. Rather, she extends her argument to consider the felt powerlessness already experienced by both caretaker and cared-for. Add to this the personal nature of the tasks involved—as Asch points out, home care aides have access to keys to the home, must handle money for shopping, must look in cupboards and drawers to find things in the home, must touch the client in transferring her from bed to wheelchair, and must often do the most intimate tasks of bathing and dressing—and one can perhaps see why Asch supports a racist client's request.

But there are other reasons for countenancing the racist's request that return to worries I raised concerning gift giving. Since our relationships are intimately tied to the formation and maintenance of our identities, we must guard against damaging relationships that rob individuals of dignity, self-respect, and positive self-concepts. Aides' rejection of gifts may have a negative effect on clients by attacking their sense of engagement with others and their identities as beings-in-relationship. The same is true of racial minorities: By placing them in positions where a negative relational dynamic is at work, such workers are put at risk of being spit at, humiliated, rejected, and stereotyped. But worse, black or Hispanic workers may feel their very identities as blacks or Hispanics are attacked and destroyed, potentially resulting in negative self-concepts caused by constant degradation. Home care relationships are not occasional or brief. They are often ongoing, and aides may spend several hours a day in contact with clients. This means that home care workers are potentially subject to long-term, racist harangues by clients who do not want nonwhite workers in their homes. To place minority workers—who are already harmed by an exploitative home care system and a broader racist culture—in such identity-crushing situations is immoral and should be avoided.

In addition, given my concerns for context, it will be difficult to differentiate one kind of client request from another. For example, as Oliver J. Williams suggests, one might be hard-put to distinguish a client's request for a white worker from a client's request for a black one. Suppose, as he suggests, that a white client would only accept a black worker, based on her view that blacks are well suited to menial tasks. Or suppose a black client would only accept black home care workers. How are we to judge the force of these requests (207–208)?

Williams pushes us to distinguish between the kinds of requests one might face by clients in the home care setting. And while I would want to distinguish a black client's request to be cared for by a black worker (based on the reasonableness of the client's concern about how she may be perceived and treated by a white home care aide), I do not think we can distinguish between the white client's request for a white worker versus her request for a black one. Both are based on racist assumptions and stereotypes; both derive from ignorance and, perhaps, fear of the "other."

Thus, when we talk about racial issues in home care, we must return to the issue of reciprocity and receiving. It is arguably immoral to reject a racist's request to have only white caretakers if the likely result will be that the care by the aide is not taken up, or received in an ethical way, by the cared-for. Clients have moral responsibilities to their aides, too. This means the degradation and humiliation of minority home care workers is also found in the rejection of their offerings of care, not just in racial prejudices or stereotypes held by the home care recipient. The harms done by pairing minority home care workers with racist clients are linked not just to racist stereotypes, then, but to the actual relationship involved and the likelihood that it will decimate the workers' sense of self-worth.[3]

However, the determination to not subject black or Hispanic workers to racist clients should not be made on their behalf. Rather, responses to racism in home care should largely be formulated by the workers who are involved in the day-to-day care. I will say much more toward the end of this chapter about the issue of communication in home care. But for now it is important to note that discourse surrounding these issues that fail to include those most centrally affected could constitute another form of racism. As Noddings points out, "The fact is that many of us have been reduced to cases by the very machinery that has been instituted to care for us" (1996, 27).

### Abuse of Clients within the Home Care Setting

One of the most distressing problems that arises in the home care context is abuse of clients by caretakers. One might think there is little to say about this issue—it's wrong, and abusive workers simply should not be tolerated. And while this is true, it is important to understand the origins of such abuse and how the home care system itself creates and perpetuates it. Abuse of vulnerable clients by home care workers (and family caretakers) represents the worst kind of violation, since it takes place within what is supposed to be the safe space of the home, where one escapes the vulnerabilities inherent to the public realm. But abusive home care relationships must be understood *in terms of* relationship, for once again objective, principled accounts of the wrongness of abuse fail to address the important relational features that lead to it. In what follows, I will consider abusive home care relationships through the feminist lens of relational autonomy to show that they are a reaction against an impersonal, exploitative, frustrating, and psychically harmful system of home health care.

One of the four major principles of health care ethics as identified by Tom Beauchamp and James Childress is the principle of non-maleficence, or "first do no harm." It is arguably a minimal principle in health care ethics because if we can't actually benefit or do good for patients, then at the very least we can refrain from harming them. And, it would seem, the principle is highly appropriate to the home care setting, too. As a venue for providing health care to people, home care may arguably be governed by the same moral considerations that attach to institutional health care provision.

But by appealing to non-maleficence in cases of client abuse in home care, we fail to see the prior harms that occurred: harms to the families and workers taking care of clients. At the organizational level of home care services, an extremely exploitative system of care is put in place, and families and formal caretakers of clients are subjected to the harsh realities of that system. It is unsurprising that, in response to their own abuse and exploitation, families and workers may pass it along to the very persons for whom they are supposed to be caring.

In a series on home health care in crisis, the *Record* (a New Jersey newspaper) indicates the serious problem of criminal caretakers, that is, individuals with a criminal record for stealing, drug dealing, and violent offenses who are working as home health aides. "In nearly every county, the *Record* found criminals—fully certified by the state—working alone in the homes of cancer survivors, the elderly, and the infirm, their pasts hidden from vulnerable patients."[4] Part of the problem of "criminal caretakers" is attributable to the conditions under which home health care is currently practiced. As I indicated in chapter 1, home care wages are notoriously low, and in a thriving economy, agencies may have difficulty recruiting good workers. Indeed, few people are willing to take on the high demands of home care work for a mere $5.56 or $7.00 per hour. The result is a pool of workers who are less than desirable, some who steal from clients or put them at serious risk through physical abuse or harmful restraint.

As just one example of the kinds of abuse at work, consider home care aide Helen Thompson, who locked a client with Alzheimer's disease in her car while she cared for another client in a house down the street. Thompson did this in August 1998, under sweltering conditions that almost caused the death of her client. It is not uncommon for home care aides to abuse not only clients but the home care system itself by double-booking for shifts with two home care agencies. In situations like Thompson's, the aide only shows up at one client's home, but bills both agencies for her time. Or the aide may confine one client (as Thompson did) in order to provide service in another client's home. The problem is that clients are often incapable of reporting the abuse, since they may have advanced Alzheimer's disease or be too fearful or concerned about losing services to report it.

However, abuse can take other forms as well. As one case study indicates, financial exploitation is another aspect of client abuse:

> Abuse cases are not always clear cut, especially when financial exploitation is at stake. The case manager has a case now in which the client's So-

cial Security check is the only regular income in the home, and her son and his family depend on it. The client is only "sometimes competent," but she is adamant that she wants to stay in that home. The family is on the neglectful side, but they say they love their mother and want her with them. The case manager believes the woman could get better care in a nursing home and that a case of financial exploitation and neglect could be made. But should it be? (Kane and Caplan, 112)

Here the ways in which clients are financially exploited—another form of abuse—becomes evident. Such abuse is not only at the hands of formal caretakers, however, but may also be visited by families themselves, who may use the client to receive necessary financial support. Clearly, while such activities are problematic, the problems go beyond caretaking to include broader concerns for a state that fails to adequately provide for its poorest members.

The other problem that leads to abuse of home care clients is the "unlicensed underground" at work in the home care industry. Since a large percentage of the nation's home care costs are paid out-of-pocket by senior citizens and their families, people are looking for affordable care solutions. Many turn to unlicensed, untrained workers who will work for a fraction of the cost of licensed help. But in so doing, they sacrifice the few protections offered by legitimate home care providers. In such cases, workers are hired through advertisements in newspapers, by word-of-mouth, or through other informal avenues. But as one owner of a home care agency puts it, "A lot of consumers don't realize the risk they're taking when they go to the underground. You have to ask yourself, 'Do you want to hire a person who would be willing to do this work for only $40 a day?'"[5]

Here a feminist critique is called for, since it is tempting to reduce these reports of abuse to evil or immoral individuals who are violating their duty of care. But such reductionism is a moral mistake. While abuse of vulnerable home care clients is, indeed, intolerable, the cause should be rooted not in the terrible judgment of a few individuals or families but in the very construction of the practice of home care. Furthermore, when we focus our vision through a feminist lens, we see the way in which negative relational dynamics can lead to abuse of clients, not only by formal caretakers but also by their own loved ones.

For the most part, this book has focused on the kinds of positive, "kinlike" relationships that home care fosters. Relationships between formal caretakers and their clients can become more like familial ones, where parties come to not only care for, but care about, one another. Yet in some cases such loving bonds are not fostered, and the relationships take on a negative dynamic that is harmful to both caretaker and client. And sometimes this negative dynamic is caused by the broader home care system, where workers are subjected to low pay, poor working conditions, lack of benefits, and an impersonal system that treats them as cogs in a machine. Under such working conditions, it is less surprising that abuse by caretakers occurs. To return to my Foucauldian point in chapter 2, relationships of power are manifest when caretakers engage in passing along to clients their abuse and exploitation by the home care system. As Foucault has shown us, such manifestations of power are the expected result of systems of power and domination.

For example, take a common scenario of a home health aide who is overworked, underpaid, without benefits, and lacking the moral support of the home care supervisors at her agency. When she calls in to report problems in her clients' homes, her concerns are passed off because the home care supervisors are burdened with heavy case loads. This leaves the aide feeling isolated, frustrated, and abandoned. Add to these difficulties a client with dementia who refuses the aide's care, struggling and screaming when she tries to wash the client. Now one can understand the dangerousness of the home care relationship. The aide's lashing out at her client is akin to her lashing out at the system itself, yet she cannot extricate herself from it because she lacks the education and training to do other kinds of work.

What I am arguing for, then, is a reconceptualization of abuses in the home care setting. While we should, indeed, act to remedy individual abuses visited by workers on their clients, our scope of concern should not end there. There are questions we must ask that implicate us *all* in such abuses, such as: What social factors led up to the client's abuse by her caretaker? Did the aide receive the necessary emotional and moral support in working through problems that arise in her home care practice? In what ways are family members isolated and abandoned such that abusive situations arise? Would psychological services help family members deal with the stresses of caretaking? And perhaps most important, we should ask: How do current social and economic conditions lend themselves to possible abuse situations in the home care setting? When we ask these broader questions, we place home care within its proper social and political context. This is the very kind of treatment of caretaking issues for which feminist theorists like Eva Kittay and Martha Fineman are arguing.

Thus, to remedy abuse problems in home care would mean changing the very basis of home care, no longer seeing it as a private, parochial problem. If caretaking needs are put in their proper social and political context, issues of fair pay and fair treatment for families and workers come to the fore, and we can get at the deeper-rooted, culture-based problems of client abuse in home care.

### Negotiating between Individual and Community

With "do no harm" as the overriding goal, protecting clients ultimately
may mean declining to serve them in their own homes because the plan
may be unsafe. (Kane and Levin, 76)

Often the most painful, and morally difficult, relational question that
arises in the home care setting is how to determine when it is no longer safe
for a client to remain in her home. Such determinations are only made more
complicated when—whether she is competent or not—the client refuses to
leave home, and the decision must be made against her will. Herein I will
pursue the question of how to negotiate such situations. Rather than strictly
relying on a principle of autonomy, however, I will again consider a feminist conception of relational autonomy that places our choices and desires
within the context of a self embedded in social relationships. A bald appeal
to autonomy is undesirable for many reasons: first, because it treats individuals in isolation from others with whom they are in relationship; second,
because sometimes the capacity for autonomy is absent or minimal in
clients, so autonomy may be elusive; and third, because an important goal
is to prevent harm to both the client and those living in community with
her. A feminist conception of relational autonomy may yield different an-
swers in different situations, but this is as it should be. When dealing with
individuals of varying competencies and social situations, we cannot derive
a simple principle like "there's no place like home."

To begin, consider the situation I experienced as a home care aide for an
elderly woman who lived alone in an apartment complex. I was brought in
to help Marguerite because she couldn't move or get out of bed without
screaming in pain. Marguerite reported to me that she had slipped on her
waxed floor after the maid had been in to clean the house, a story that
seemed believable until her daughter-in-law told me that Marguerite had no
maid. Her children were frustrated by their inability to deal with their
mother. She was starting to smell because she couldn't get up for a bath, she
needed proper genital care, and she had been lying in the same nightgown
for days on end. Family members were afraid to move Marguerite for fear
of harming her. Furthermore, because of work pressures, they weren't able
to stay with her around the clock. My job was to get Marguerite out of
bed, bathe her and ensure she successfully completed her toileting, and
make meals for her. Her daughter-in-law warned me that Marguerite had
been preparing her own meals, then putting dirty cutlery and dishes back
in the cupboards. Another part of my job, then, was to return her apartment to order, including washing all the dishes in her cupboards and re-

moving the soiled toilet tissue that Marguerite had been throwing in the bathtub instead of the toilet.

At first, getting Marguerite out of bed was a terrifying process. As she had no medical equipment in her home (like a wheelchair for mobility), I pulled a kitchen chair up to her bedside and transferred her from bed to chair. Since her apartment floors were hardwood, I was able to slide the chair around the apartment with her on it to spare her the seemingly painful activity of walking from room to room. I would count to three to prepare Marguerite to be moved, and when I did the transfer she would cry and moan. Once settled on the chair, however, she appeared comfortable, and I was able to help with her bathing and dressing.

Marguerite was a sweet and charming woman. She had many stories about her homeland and what it was like growing up. But most of the time she was confused and frightened; she had the paranoid delusion that men were coming into her apartment and stealing her jewelry. Given these circumstances, I was sick with worry every time I left her alone. The arrangement had been made that when my shift was over, I would use Marguerite's key to lock the apartment and then hang the key under the wreath on her door. It deeply concerned me that this client was locked inside her apartment alone, yet I alone could not provide the 24-hour care that she really needed, as I was in graduate school at the time and had other clients to care for.

One morning when I came off the elevator to Marguerite's apartment, I found her wandering down her hallway, banging on people's doors and crying for help. I helped her back to her apartment and found that, in her confused state, she had dragged the kitchen table all the way to the doorway of her apartment. She had managed to unlock her door from the inside and, in her panic, begun pounding on doors to call for help. It was inconceivable to me that this tiny woman, who screamed in pain when I tried to sit her up or move her, had got out of bed on her own, dragged a heavy table to the door (which served no purpose in her escape), and run down the hallway.

In short, I was very uneasy about Marguerite remaining in her home alone. As a mere home care aide, I had no input into her competency to remain at home, as this was considered a question to be settled by mental status tests and psychiatrists, not by an aide who helped her perform her activities of daily living. Yet it was clear to me that Marguerite was a danger to both herself and her neighbors. She did not have enough clarity of mind to be alone in her home, and it was conceivable that she might leave burners turned on or somehow start a fire. But Marguerite *knew* that she was home, and her family knew that removing her would prove difficult.

Though paranoid and deluded at times, she was aware of her environment, and she would not consider removal to a care facility.

I relate this particular case because it addresses some of the relational issues that arise when considering whether a client should remain in her home. I wish to leave aside economic questions regarding the costs of keeping someone like Marguerite at home, and consider the moral question of when this goal is appropriate.[6] As I will contend, the only ethical way to make this determination is via a relational ethic that is sensitive to the relationships at risk.

Robin Fiore criticizes gerontological ethics for the way in which the elderly individual's interest in personal autonomy is measured by her relationship to family and friends and balanced against the autonomy of formal caretakers and agencies. As she claims,

> On this view, an agent's essential interest in the maintenance of personal integrity is rendered as on par with other agents' interests in acting without constraint for convenience and profit. More importantly, characterizing the concern as a matter of justice completely obscures the central ethical issue: Those with the power to determine what counts as the appropriate compromise operate under financial incentives to provide care in forms that undermine the care recipient's autonomy and ultimately her health and well-being. (246)

Fiore is right that it is morally wrong to subject an individual's basic interests to fiscal considerations. As I will argue in chapter 6, as a community we need to determine a standard of care that considers what level of care a decent society should provide, how we are to provide it, and how those who do provide it will be treated. And this should be done prior to questions about how much we have to spend on it. But I reject Fiore's claim that it is immoral to place the individual home care client's wishes in the context of her relationship to others. An individual's interest in remaining at home should not be viewed as a "trump card" that he can play, one that outweighs all other considerations (like the potential for him to harm others if he remains at home, or his own safety). Rather, such requests—or demands—are rightly viewed in terms of accommodation, not autonomy. Insofar as it is possible, one's desire to remain at home for as long as possible should be accommodated, especially when one's self-concepts, sense of place, and relationships with others are connected to home. But given my home care experiences with individuals like Marguerite, I do not think that a traditional appeal to autonomy addresses the complex moral issues that are involved.

Since part of my concern is with the way in which our very selves are constituted by our relationships with others, an important consideration in a case like Marguerite's is the impact that removal from her home will have on her self-understandings and her agency. Indeed, some degree of agency was still apparent in Marguerite—for example, she was capable of expressing her desire to be at home—and it would be insensitive to reduce for convenience's sake the degree to which she was capable of making self-regarding choices. So an important question on my feminist approach is how the move from home to long-term care institution would affect the client.

Essentially, the concerns raised when a client wishes to remain at home relate to acceptable degrees of risk for both client and caretakers. Furthermore, we have to be clear about what *kind* of risk is at stake. Do we mean merely physical risks (for example, of falling, burning down the apartment building, putting others at risk), or do we include psychological or social risks? As I see it, the psycho-social risks are at least as important as physical ones and should be accounted for when one attempts to answer these difficult questions. It is a relevant concern that a client, who is still capable of identifying self with home, may be torn from that supportive moral and ontological space.[7]

Rosalie Kane and Carrie Levin have addressed risk-taking in home care and have offered some elements that ought to be considered when appraising acceptable risk levels. These elements include type of risk (physical, psychological, social), severity of consequences, likelihood of consequences, difficulty of predicting risk, negative effects of avoiding the risk, and the role of providers (78–79). What I like most about their approach is their appreciation of the relational aspect of these considerations. For example, the authors recognize that we are sometimes balancing the client's willingness to accept a risk against the caretaker's reluctance to engage in a relationship where someone for and about whom she cares might be harmed. And sometimes we are weighing an individual's choice (to be at home and risk falling, for example) against considerations of how likely it is that the bad effect will occur.

Kane and Levin suggest one way of dealing with a client's desire to remain in the home versus others' desire that she be placed elsewhere: managed risk contracting. As they explain it, such contracting involves parties coming together to iron out a contract indicating what risks the client is willing to take and to legally absolve providers of responsibility. As they state,

> Ultimately, the person incurring the risk is perceived as the ultimate decision-maker (assuming competency and no inordinate risks to others), but the search is always for compromise solutions. The plan is documented in writing and signed by the consumer and other parties relevant to the agreement. (79)

This solution may appear to be a solid response to the relational concerns I have been raising. Managed risk contracting may allow for the kind of communicative give-and-take for which I have been arguing, and it may seem to provide for an individual who strongly identifies with home to stay there. But I reject this recent trend in dealing with these important relational problems. For it merely extends the received view of individuals as contracting parties who are coming together for mutual benefit and protection. And turning complex relationships of care into the occasion for social contract entirely misses the feminist point. For while parties may be able to contract away their legal obligations to one another, they surely cannot contract away their moral ones. As a moral subject and a home care aide, my concerns for particular clients would not have been eliminated by the existence of a contract releasing me (or my agency) from legal responsibility for them.

Nevertheless, Kane and Levin are right that others' predictions of risk, no matter how unlikely, should not be used as automatic grounds for dismissing the client's desire to remain at home. "Often," they say, "professionals and family members of the older person with the disability concentrate on the severity of consequences, say, if an older person with some dementia is alone in the home and becomes prey to a dangerous criminal, rather than concentrating on the likelihood of such an event actually occurring" (78).

To put my position succinctly, we need to consider "risk" in its broadest possible sense, including the risks inherent to pulling individuals out of their homes and communities. This type of risk is not given enough of our attention and is one thing that a feminist relational approach highlights and that other approaches tend to overlook. We should be willing to countenance the possibility that a client (who is capable of making the determination) may place psycho-social risks above physical ones, meaning that she is willing to stay in her home to prevent the harms associated with relocation, even if that means she is at risk of falling when she is home alone. Some clients may indeed value their relationships—with home, with caretakers, with friends and neighbors—more than their physical safety.

And what of clients like Marguerite, who are capable neither of the kind of managed risk contracting that Kane and Levin present nor of making the clear determination that they wish to remain at home? The answer as to whether or not they should remain at home is found in a variety of factors: Whether the client has expressed some desire to be there, whether the continued home placement allows for decent care for the individual,[8] and whether continued placement in their homes will allow for the continuation of relationships that are of moral significance to the client.[9]

As for Marguerite herself, she was eventually transferred to the only place available at the time: the local psychiatric hospital. Her family was extremely saddened by this move, partly because of the implications for their relationship with her, and partly because of the conditions under which she had to live there. And I felt the loss of her as a client, though I do think the choice to leave her at home would have been a highly problematic one.

### Family Caretaking: To Pay or Not to Pay?

The issue of paid family caretaking has been recently debated in home care literature.[10] Unsurprisingly, the practice engenders strong responses both in favor of and against it: Supporters claim that it provides some payment for and recognizes work done by family members; detractors argue that it leads to exploitation and abuse of both the home care client and the agencies themselves.

My own position on this topic is conflicted, and as a result, my response to the question of whether to pay family members for caretaking is multilayered. On the one hand, in line with my earlier critiques of the perversion of the care ethic, I resent the state's exploitation of women by calling on their free care work for loved ones. Payment for this labor is desirable, as is the resulting recognition that it *is* labor. On the other hand, where this practice has been implemented, family members have been poorly paid, meaning that such minimal payments may only further the exploitation of family in service of the state.

I have two responses to the question of paid family caretaking, and they address two levels of concern. When considering this practice from within the current framework of home care provision, I support the remuneration of family members for the care work that they do. That is, as an affirmative remedy,[11] paid family caretaking is a supportable policy. But this system of payment will still be occurring within a gendered division of labor, guided by individualism and connected to the contractualist notion of relationships. So on the level of radical change, in isolation of other major social changes, such a policy fails. In chapter 6 I will consider the ideal social and political conditions under which home care should be practiced and will thus develop my call for a more radical project. For now, let us consider the ethics of paid family caretaking within the current home care context. Again, with consideration for issues in relational autonomy, I will argue for the ethical propriety of such payments.

Jean Blaser cites important worries related to its implementation, including (1) exploitation (such a policy "exploits family values by paying the family member less than the going 'market' rate for provided services"), (2) the potential for fraud and abuse (since family members have tended to defraud and/or abuse clients and programs), (3) increased administrative costs (since extra measures are required to investigate abuses of clients and systems), and (4) increased program costs (since families will supposedly scramble to sign up for reimbursement for caretaking). While all these problems are serious indeed, my moral concerns focus especially on the potential exploitation and the increased program costs that are likely to result from paid family caretaking. Blaser expresses concern about the exploitation of paid family caretakers. As she argues, family members may agree to accept such employment because they cannot find a nonfamily worker. Indeed, family members will give up the opportunity to receive higher wages in the workforce for the sake of their loved ones. Blaser worries that such arrangements merely continue exploitation and remove incentives for social change (66).

Yet as real as these concerns are, and as poor an option as paid family caretaking may be, the alternatives are worse. By refusing to consider this scheme, we condemn women to an ongoing lack of remuneration (of any kind) for their labor. What the paid caretaking option offers may not be satisfactory, but until the deeper changes occur for which I petition in chapter 6, some steps must be taken to remedy the state's free riding on familial care work.

Blaser also argues that paying family members to do care work will prevent broader changes in the home care system. Yet I am not convinced that this is true. Affirmative reform strategies like this one could conceivably transform perspectives and lead to more radical change; affirmative and transformative strategies are not mutually exclusive. On the contrary, David Ingram argues that the two are dialectical: They interact and inform one another. As he asks,

> Can we achieve transformative ends using affirmative means? Perhaps. Take the example of multicultural education. While it certainly promotes the mutual affirmation of distinct and diverse cultures, it does so only by encouraging their mutual communication; and that communication, in turn, sets in motion a process of mutual transformation whereby each informs the other, so to speak. (2000, 47)

Thus, it is not obvious that attempting to reform the current system, in part through the inception of paid family caretaking, cannot lead to broader changes. If we recognize the value of care labor by paying for it, then we may become aware of it as essential to the reproduction of our lives.

Through such a policy, we may begin to see caretaking as a social problem, not something to be left up to private individuals.

Next, consider Blaser's objection that paid family caretaking leads to exploitation and abuse of clients and providers, and that this results in increased administrative costs. Again, she is right that the circumstances under which the job is being performed—outside the public eye, where violations of the public trust and abuses of the cared-for can occur—are problematic. But this is true of home care services in any case and not just in the case of family caretakers. Abuses by paid, nonfamilial caretakers already take place in home care, so the worries about abuse and exploitation are not unique to the family. As supporters of paid family caretaking argue, "The 'family fraud' view also tends to overlook existing fraud and abuse among agency workers" (Simon-Rusinowitz et al., 74). Problems of fraud and abuse attach to the deeper moral difficulties that the practice of home care engenders. I will say more about these difficulties in chapter 6.

Finally, consider the interesting claim Blaser makes, what I will call the "out of the woodwork" objection: that if the state allows for remuneration of family caretakers, people will be crawling out of the woodwork to lay claim to such monies. As she argues, "It is not too difficult to imagine . . . a significant number of families applying for the benefit once they learn of it" (68). Yet consider this response to Blaser's worry: that if we are going to institute such a policy, and these individuals are, indeed, caring for elderly family members, then they are deserving of the benefit, increased program costs be damned. As I suggested earlier, we should not be deciding how much we have to spend on care for citizens and then determining whether to pay caretakers; rather, we should be determining if it is morally required of us and then go about deciding how to fund the payments.

While I am highly sympathetic to Blaser's concerns, especially as they address some of my feminist worries about the practice of home care, I disagree with her that paid family caretaking is an undesirable social policy. As an affirmative remedy for current social wrongs, it is at least a start toward recognizing the value of women's (familial) labor. And given the dialectical nature of affirmative and transformative remedies, as Ingram characterizes them, it is possible that such an affirmative remedy can lead to more transformative changes in how we value care work.

All of what I have said thus far presumes communication between parties. In order to work out these relational difficulties, people in relationship with one another must be able to talk through their differences. Yet how are we to effect this and ensure good, inclusive, moral communication? The next section will consider issues of discourse in the home care setting.

## Can We Talk? Discourse Ethics and Home Care

An increasingly utilized approach to ethics is one that was initially voiced by critical theorist Jürgen Habermas: communicative ethics.[12] In what follows, I will explore this approach and its implications for the provision of home care in particular. Both its similarities to and differences from other often-used theories (most notably, deontological, consequentialist, and feminist theories) will be indicated, and the importance this ethic places on rational democratic dialogue in the home care setting will be emphasized. Despite its difficulties, communicative ethics has much to offer a discussion of ethics and home care, from the macrolevel of policymaking to the microlevel of the individual client.

At its root, communicative ethics is concerned with ensuring the democratic participation of all members of a community, safeguarding each individual's opportunity to agree to and accept the conditions under which rational discourse takes place. A discourse "community" according to this ethic can be understood as localized (that is, a relatively small group of people living in a certain district) or any group of persons whose interests impact one another (which could include an entire state or country). Discourses at the smaller grassroots level—for example, parent-teacher associations or neighborhood watch organizations—are particularly important in that "it is hoped that such discourses will generate an autonomous and critical public opinion aimed at radicalizing discussion regarding generalizable interests at the party-politics level" (Ingram 1990, 145). In essence, then, communicative ethics aims at vocalizing the real interests of individuals that are identified through fair and impartial discussion and that result in rational agreement on issues of common interest. On this account ethics is social activity, where decision making is done by the community and where the process by which the community comes to a consensus is as important as the moral consensus itself.

Habermas's communicative ethics shares the deontologist's commitments to universalizability and reason. Like Immanuel Kant, then, Habermas claims that "under the moral point of view, one must be able to test whether a norm or a mode of action could be generally accepted by those affected by it, such that their acceptance would be rationally motivated and hence uncoerced" (1989–90, 36). Autonomy and universalizability are of central importance for Habermas in that we cannot abandon autonomous agents to societal norms or "modes of action" and in that we must test the general acceptability of (i.e., we must be able to universalize) the norm in question.

But Habermas differs from Kant in many important respects. According to Kant, the process of autonomy development is private and independent; individuals do not need others for autonomous thought and decision making, since we can rely on reason and universalizability to guide us. Indeed, on Kant's model, we must rather "block out" the others with whom we are in relationship in order to come to a rational, autonomous, impartial, reflective decision. Habermas, by contrast, asserts that the development of autonomy is social and occurs only within community. It is not a private undertaking. Autonomy develops through community, not in spite of it. Furthermore, Kant claims that the only moral actions are those that are universalizable (that is, actions whose maxims can be willed consistently as a universal law). According to him we are never to be influenced by our mere inclinations when judging morally appropriate action. On the contrary, we must fight those inclinations by applying the constraints of reason and duty. Our preferences, desires, and needs must not enter into the critical evaluation of our maxims because they are biased and partial. So, for example, a client's attitude to her caretaker should not be based on her preferences (that she doesn't want a woman of color in her home), since she would be failing to universalize her maxim and because she would not be respecting the autonomy of her caretaker. The client's needs and her inclination to act upon them are illegitimate, according to Kant, because they are subjective. Habermas, by contrast, views our preferences as a necessary part of our moral discourse because they reflect, and are reflected by, our community. In other words, we must include preferences and needs within the communicative ethic because our needs are part of our ethical lives. How we interpret our needs is determined by our ethical life and, like our principles and maxims, should be subjected to rational moral deliberation. And when we deliberate about our needs, we may accept or reject them based on the potential benefits or harms to our community, as determined by the community through the process of discussion and communication. This means that the racist client's preferences will not necessarily be respected. Whether they will be accepted or not comes out of discussion and communication of all relevant parties.

Notice that, like Kant, Habermas gives us a procedural account of ethics. What matters is the procedure or the process by which we identify needs and norms. But this is not to say that Habermas's communicative ethic lacks any concern for or interest in consequences.

Habermas's claim that we must subject our needs to rational moral deliberation, and that we will accept or reject those needs based on harms or benefits to our community, resembles a traditional consequentialist approach. According to Habermas, in evaluating needs and norms we are trying to reach consensus. The reason we agree to norms is because we evaluate our lifestyles and revise them to create the best form of life, a form of life which emerges through community discourse. As David Ingram expresses it,

> The ultimate aim of a communication ethic, then, is to bring about conditions of rational participatory democracy, in which existing needs can be critically assessed and transformed. For only by publicly discussing our needs can we begin to assess their impact on the lives of others. And, only by assessing their impact on the lives of others, can we determine their rationality, or compatibility with the general interest of all concerned. (1990, 147)

There is a noticeable concern for consequences in Habermas's demand that we assess our needs and their "impact on the lives of others." The reasonableness and rationality of our needs is at least partially dependent on whether, as Ingram puts it, they are compatible with the general interest of all concerned. So although communicative ethics is largely concerned with the process by which consensus about our norms and needs is achieved (a deontological concern), there is also consideration of the impact that the fulfillment of our needs has on the lives of others, and a focus on maximizing community values as determined through rational community discourse (consequentialist considerations).

The norms and needs that regulate a community's life are not highly abstract, then, but are the actual norms and needs as identified by individuals within the community. While some of the principles we appeal to may remain abstract—such as "respect for individual rights"—communicative ethics, like feminist ethics, is concerned with real members of the community in their lived conditions. And although Habermas does appeal to the notion of an ideal community that is made up of individuals who are participating in dialogue with all necessary knowledge, he does not suggest that this is how we actually are. This idealized conception is rather to make individuals involved in dialogue with others consider the conditions under which others find themselves and to "assume reflexive role-distance and the ability and willingness to take the standpoint of others involved in a controversy into account and reason from their point of view" (Benhabib 1996a, 76). Thus, communicative ethics is also like feminist ethics in that it accounts for oppression by differentiating fair, rational democratic discourse from ideological, oppressive discourse. Like feminist ethicists, Habermas also refuses to treat our emotional lives as private, but treats them as important to, and indeed part of, our public dialogue and laws. Unlike deontology and consequentialism, then, communicative ethics sees the emotional aspect of our lives as integral and necessary to our public dialogue. On

Habermas's view, the public/private distinction that has separated our "private" lives (including our emotions and all aspects of domestic life) from our "public" lives (work and politics) must be continually revised in discourse. What is "private" and "public" is not given but changes through dialogue.

Consider the previous cases I cited and the way a Habermasian communicative ethic can help resolve at least some of the problems that arise. Gift giving, racism, abuse, placement of clients, and paid family caretaking are all problems that are best morally addressed through inclusive, honest, and fair conversation. We could determine what ought to be done in these cases by appealing to different features of them. For example, we could focus on autonomy and argue that a client's desire to remain in her home should be respected at all times (a deontological view); we could attempt to secure the best possible outcomes by determining which action will maximize the values of all people involved (a consequentialist view); or we could highlight the power imbalances between the client and her care provider. All three of these approaches raise valid considerations, but what they miss is the importance of communication and critical conversation between individuals within a community (in this case, the "community" being the client, her family, neighbors, aides, and all the other staff involved in her care). What communicative ethics highlights is the breakdown of rational moral deliberation, the lack of democratic discussion or discourse when it appears, and a lack of sensitivity to each community member's viewpoint in coming to a consensus about norms and needs.

Habermas states the conditions necessary for rational democratic discourse as follows:

> (3.1) Every subject with the competence to speak and act is allowed to take part in the discourse.
> (3.2) a. Everyone is allowed to question any assertion whatsoever.
> b. Everyone is allowed to introduce any assertion whatsoever into the discourse.
> c. Everyone is allowed to express his attitudes, desires, and needs.
> (3.3) No speaker may, by internal or external coercion, be prevented from exercising his rights as laid down in (3.1) and (3.2). (1990, 86)

These guidelines are helpful in considering the importance of inclusive, rational discourse in the home care setting. In addressing the racist client who refuses a black caretaker, I argued that the client's demand should be considered, but that discussion and good communication would be required.

But the discourse should not exclude, for example, the black women who work for the agency and who may have their own perspectives on such client requests. For example, by assuming on behalf of these workers that they would not want to be subjected to abusive treatment by their clients, the agency fails to address the real needs and preferences of the workers; rather, their needs and preferences are imputed to them. Suppose for a moment that some black workers are willing to risk possible abuse in entering the homes of racist clients in the hopes that, once those clients meet and know women of color, their attitudes will change. Only by listening to the aides' own perspectives can these possibilities come to the fore. Indeed, Oliver J. Williams claims that "culturally proficient" home care agencies

> conduct research on issues of multi-cultural service delivery and encourage staff to openly discuss experiences in multi-cultural encounters. . . . Agency policies are but one factor in gaining cultural proficiency. . . . Practices need to become flexible and culturally impartial, and every level of the agency must participate in this process. (208–209)

Now that we have explored the basic tenets of communicative ethics, it is worthwhile to consider some criticisms of this approach. Like deontology, consequentialism, and feminist ethics, communicative ethics is not without its problems. Interestingly, although communicative ethics shares many of the commitments of feminist ethics, it is largely feminist ethicists who have criticized this approach.[13] Most of these criticisms question the notions of "reason" and "rational discourse" that are foundational to communicative ethics.

One criticism of communicative ethics is that appealing to reason can ultimately exclude those who do not conform to the ideal rational model. Take, for example, a woman who wants to remain in her home at great personal physical risk. The reasons she gives may not reflect the model of rational deliberation that has been set out by Habermas. While she may offer an account of her deliberations, to outsiders her account may seem nonsensical because her needs cannot be expressed in propositional language. She may offer a personal narrative that does not appeal to moral principles and/or "objective" evidence accepted by all; as a result, her reasons may appear to some members of the community not to be reasons at all. Habermas's reliance on a conception of "rational" deliberation results in the potential exclusion of individuals within the community, which goes against the very democratic communicative ethic that he is trying to develop.

A second criticism relates to the concern about individuals who do not reason according to the ideal rational model. Critics of communicative ethics ask the further question: What is "rational" discourse? Who determines what counts as such? The norms for rational discourse are relative to different groups within our culture. So, for example, a Native American discourse that is based on a conception of the earth as a living organism may appear irrational to individuals who are not members of that community. Although communicative ethics does require that we question the very norms that are the bases for our conversations, we are still working within a norm of rational discourse. To consider an example in the realm of home care, imagine an Asian family who refuses to do what the home care agency considers to be the right thing: fully palliating their elderly mother. The family explains that their mother values clarity of mind, and that for religious reasons it is important that she meet her pain bravely, and free of painkillers, before she dies. For some community members steeped in the practice of western medicine, this discourse may seem foreign and, perhaps, irrational: they can make no sense of allowing clients to suffer. The conception of "rational" discourse, then, proves problematic, since we would first have to decide what constitutes rational discourse and who determines what counts as such.

The third critique of communicative ethics concerns the aim of discourse. Recall the earlier point that, according to Habermas, in evaluating needs and norms we are trying to reach consensus. But should the aim of discourse be to reach consensus or to express differences? Shouldn't we worry about glossing over relevant differences between community members? If the aim is to reach consensus through a rational, democratic procedure, then people may be constrained by the goal and forced to put aside differences that may be important to the discourse. A good way of understanding this problem is in terms of assimilation, where individuals from other cultures are expected to assimilate to western cultural traditions. In so doing, those individuals are being told to put aside differences in order to stay in synch with western laws, practices, and ethics. But this assimilationist view glosses over some very important cultural differences that should not be ignored, especially if we are to have a fair and democratic community discourse. The criticism of reaching consensus is analogous to the criticism of assimilation: The very aim of consensus leads us to focus on similarities between community members to the detriment of important differences within the community that must be accounted for.

These criticisms raise some fairly serious worries about communicative ethics: We cannot ignore them. But this does not render communicative ethics unusable in home care practice, any more than the problems with deontology, consequentialism, or feminist ethics render those theories worthless or unusable. Despite its problems, communicative ethics understands the core ethical enterprise to be a fair, clear, democratic discourse that will allow each individual's needs to surface; this conception of ethics has much to offer the practice of home care, since fair, democratic discourse is imperative to its being done well.

### Conclusion

In this chapter, I outlined some ethical issues that arise in personal relationships between clients and caretakers. As the chapter title suggests, though the problems are experienced on a personal level, "the personal is political"— meaning that we must place these parochial problems in the context of broader moral issues in home health care. Abuse and exploitation of clients, for example, is indeed a difficult personal situation between caretakers and clients. But as I argued, such abuses are connected to macro-level problems of home care, where caretakers are exploited by poor pay, lack of benefits, and little to no recognition for the value of their work. So, too, when we consider issues of gift giving, the ethical issue may appear to be only a personal one ("Should I accept the gift or not?") until we broaden our perspective to consider feminist concerns for reciprocity and respect.

I ended this chapter with a discussion of communicative ethics and home health care. This is a crucial issue, since good home care practice is dependent on the quality of communicative practices between parties in the home care enterprise. Many of the serious moral problems I encountered in my own practice arose because there was no forum for communicating perspectives, worries, and needs. A communicative ethics approach is particularly useful to home care because it calls for inclusive and democratic conversation, from the most empowered community members (representatives from the home care agency) to the most marginalized ones (home care aides and clients).

The final chapter will bring together the critiques I have offered thus far and will consider what home care would look like under ideal social and political conditions. While some critics will charge me with a certain utopianism, I respond that we need to be able to imagine things otherwise. It is through the power of imagination that we conceive of practices as they could be and should be, without being curtailed by how things are in their current state. Yes, managed care is the current paradigm under which home care is practiced, and critics may claim that the ethicist's job is to consider ethical issues from within that paradigm. Kathryn Christiansen asks, "How can a . . . home care agency position itself to take advantage of the managed care paradigm?" (115). But I am not interested in this question, since it involves a capitulation to the managed care model. Furthermore, as feminist theorist Catriona Mackenzie has asserted, "One way in which oppressive social relationships and institutions may impair autonomy is by restricting agents' imaginative repertoires" (124). By failing to consider how things might be otherwise, then, ethicists may very well fail in their moral obligation to think outside the box; and it may well be a sign that, with such impaired imaginative repertoires, we are no longer fit to do the job.

# 6 Looking Ahead

*Can Home Care Be Reformed?*

     This chapter is perhaps the most important in this book. It lays the grounds for what I take to be a minimally decent system of home health care. In light of the criticisms I have leveled against home care in its current condition, I will herein consider what needs to be done to make the home care enterprise an ethical one. The arguments I construct will come from two marginalized critical perspectives: Marxism and feminism. From a Marxist perspective, I will consider the limits of markets in health care and home care; I will also consider the way that value has been constructed so that noncapitalist means of producing and reproducing human life (through women's reproduction, childcare, and care of society's dependents) have been devalued and obscured. In a capitalist economy, women's care work becomes virtually nonexistent because it is "nonproductive" work, and this, I will argue, is part of the problem. Second, from a feminist perspective I will consider the moral limits of our current system of home care, where the care that is offered to clients is entirely dependent upon our economic ability (and willingness) to put money toward such care. As I will argue, we have done a kind of moral reversal in the way that home care services are

viewed: Instead of seeing ourselves as a moral community with certain obligations to care for one another, we see ourselves as an economic entity
with prior economic obligations that limit how much we are willing to spend
on care. From these two marginal perspectives, I will indicate why the current manifestation of home care is immoral and why transformation, and
not just affirmative reform strategies, should be the ultimate goal for ethicists and home care policymakers.

### Alienation, Value, and Markets in Home Care

To begin with my Marxist concerns, consider the practice of home
care within our current capitalist system. In treating home care, one cannot
divorce it from the broader problems created by the U.S. system of managed care. Some of my comments, then, will refer directly to the organization of home care, and some will refer to the general provision of health
care. Furthermore, my critical position is not dependent on the kind of
"revolution" with which Marxists are generally disparagingly associated,
for while I do think that serious class-based inequalities need to be rectified,
my account of the required transformations in our provision of care is not
reliant upon a broader social revolution. In this, I concur with Milton Fisk's
assertion that "there is the option . . . of moving a few sectors at a time
with a political program for transforming them in accord with similar general aims. This contrasts with the option of focusing from the outset on
changing the foundations of the society as a whole" (187).

Consider the problems associated with home care as it is practiced within a market-based system of health care. Home care workers are alienated in
the classical Marxist sense. On Marx's critique, all workers under capitalism
are alienated, as we are all separated from the things we are creating and exploited in their production. Since, for Marx, we are what we make, alienation
is caused by both our part in the production of meaningless objects, as well
as our estrangement from our work as we reproduce our "species-being."

But care workers are doubly alienated by their work and life conditions.
That is, they are held to the general expectation that they will care for and
about their clients; yet the home care system is set up in such a way as to
block the authentic expression of care. What makes the process worse is
that the organization of home care separates the very things that make
home care workers human—the moral capacity to care—from their work,
while at the same time invoking their care for others as the grounds for
paying them badly. The result is an incoherence in the system, crazy-
making for workers doing the menial jobs, and, ultimately, alienation of the
worst kind.

I cited examples in chapter 2 that relate to this concern for alienation. Care plans that reduce the work done by aides to washing and dressing bodies and feeding mouths, scarcely giving them enough time to complete the bare mechanics of these acts, turn them into "instruments" in the care of clients. Under such conditions, one could characterize the home care "aide" as an "aid"; rather than being viewed by the organization as a human being providing physical *and* moral care to clients, she becomes a mere instrument—like a hoyer lift or an electric wheelchair—that provides the mechanical support needed by the client.

In her essay "Life's Work," Vicki Schultz argues that working women fare better than nonworking ones:

> Research clearly shows that work offers women a chance for heightened self-esteem, a buffer against depression, and enhanced mental and physical health. And this isn't just true for women in high-powered jobs. Working-class women get the emotional and physical benefits of working. (1909)

Yet often in home care, workers are denied the beneficial aspects of their work by virtue of the market context within which it is taking place. Workers receive opposing messages: that their work should be a "labor of love," and because of that, they aren't deserving of fair pay for it; and that they should avoid emotional attachment to their clients and view their caretaking as instrumentally (and not intrinsically) valuable. Schultz's claim that paid work has positive health effects on women, then, fails to account for the emotional, mental, and physical trauma experienced by low-paid home care workers.[1]

I locate other alienating aspects of home care work in the capitalist system of value by which home care is judged. A capitalist economy appropriates women's unremunerated and badly remunerated labor, making it socially and economically invisible and, thus, nonexistent. Home care is construed as "nonproductive" work, since it involves the relentless and repetitive tasks that are associated with the activities of daily living. Even physicians, who are engaged in a different form of cultural production—the production of healthy bodies—can be said to "produce" citizens who are supposedly brought from a nonfunctioning, nonproductive state to a healthy, normal one where they can return to capitalist activities of production. In our current value system, home care aides fail to do even this much, as the clients with whom they are dealing are not likely to be returned to a state of productivity. Thus, within a capitalist schema, home care aides appear to be nonproductive.

The value of home care services to individuals who give and receive them should be distinguished conceptually from the value of home care services within a capitalist state. Clearly, individuals benefit from and value the care services they receive, since care allows them to stay at home. Caretaking services even have economic value to the state, since, as I argued in chapter 1, by transferring the costs of caring to individual families, the state extracts economic value from familial labor. But the economic value of home care is directly dependent on its continued social *de*valuation, such that there is a vested state interest in not socially valuing it. The low social value of home care work and the continued economic value of it are necessarily connected: the less socially valued the care work, the less remuneration is due to those who engage in it. The lowlier and less educated the labor pool, the less payment is required for their services. Thus, I am pessimistic that change in the way we conceive of care work will come easily, since there are corporate and capitalist reasons for not wanting such conceptual change to occur.

For these reasons, I argue that health care (and, by extension, home health care) should be moved out of the for-profit sector, rather than waiting for change in our social valuation of care work. There are both moral and economic arguments for this move. Morally speaking, a market system of health care treats health as a commodity to be bought and sold on the market, and this in turn treats patients as health care "consumers" in the most literal sense. Such a conception of patients glosses over the deep inequalities between consumers who purchase widgets on the market and patients who must seek health care services from a care provider. Consumers may access information regarding the widgets they are purchasing that is simply not available to patients who are "shopping around" for a good thoracic surgeon. A market model of health care also serves to commodify health, something which is arguably so basic to human flourishing and one's ability to be "productive" that it does not fit well with market goals. Markets in BMWs are one thing; markets in health care are another.

The economic argument for shifting health care out of the for-profit sector rests on the amount of government monies committed to running a health care system that suffers from corporate bloat. As Robert Kuttner points out,

> The market aspects of the American health-care system impose immense, unnecessary administrative costs absent in a universal system. These include, first, a far greater degree of paperwork. The fastest-growing category of health-care job is claims clerk. Since there is no standard form or standard plan, each insurer has its own rules, reimbursement procedures, and formulas. (146)

Many commentators have argued against the waste and incoherence associated with markets in medicine. Since this book is on home health care and is not a critique of health care in general, I cannot pursue these critiques in detail. But inasmuch as the broader system of health care dictates the provision of home care services, we need to be clear that any discussion of home care change necessarily points to changes in the provision of health care generally. And while critics argue that *all* systems of health care provision are flawed, including fee-for-service and universal health care, managed care is a particularly flawed and pernicious mode of providing health care to citizens. I see little hope of making home health care just if it continues to be provided within the context of managed care.

Moreover, both the state and big business have prevented the kind of Marxist class consciousness that could lead to change in the provision of health care. While managed care is, in some sense, based on a conception of patients as part of a collective (since physicians must decide what services to offer to a particular patient while bearing in mind the impact on her entire patient population), there is no real encouragement of shared needs and interests. As Marxists point out, once a consciousness develops of individuals as part of a class of people with shared interests and experiences, then we may develop a class consciousness that demands the kind of health care reform not desired by those with an interest in the status quo.

The same avoidance of class consciousness is apparent in the home care industry. One need only imagine the social and economic undesirability of care workers developing a sense of their oppression and exploitation as a class. In developing this sense, workers may begin to demand better wages, better working conditions, and decent benefits. Indeed, as I will discuss, the home care industry has already been affected by this consciousness-raising, as home care workers are unionizing in increasing numbers. This unionizing has occurred despite practices and policies that isolate workers and that prevent the opportunities for discourse between and among them.[2]

As I see it, the attempts to unionize and democratize home care must be taken up by workers themselves, which means that somehow barriers to their self-organization must be overcome. As Penny Hollander Feldman has indicated,

> Scattered across multiple work sites, home-care workers are far more difficult to unionize than health-care workers in institutional settings. The vast majority of professional and paraprofessional employees do not belong to unions. Nevertheless, in some large cities, unions have successfully organized the aide workforce principally in agencies that contract with state and local governments to provide publicly financed services. (160)

Organizing for change proves difficult for home care workers because of their isolation from one another. For example, in my years as a home care aide, I seldom met or spoke with other aides. My one-week training took place at my home care office, where I trained with other newly hired workers. But as new recruits we had no sense of what the job would be like, that we might want to exchange names and telephone numbers, or that we might need to organize to protect our rights as workers. And while aides are often required to attend "in-services," where new home care techniques or safety procedures are taught, these in-services do not permit much interaction. Finally, interaction outside the home care agency proves almost impossible, as aides never work together on shifts, and work schedules vary greatly. Opportunities for sharing experiences, oppressions, and ideas are minimal, thus making the development of class consciousness extremely difficult.

Since home care work is rooted in the private sphere of the home rather than the sphere of public institutions, one could easily argue that working conditions only accidentally prevent aides from organizing. It is unavoidable and inevitable, one could argue, that home care workers are isolated from one another. I recognize that this is true, but would add that disciplining practices within the home care industry are designed to further alienate worker from client and worker from worker. Home care work not only fails to build solidarity; it is designed to actively prevent worker solidarity from occurring. From a Foucauldian perspective, home care is organized such that individual workers and clients become disciplined to the regulations, procedures, and practices governing its delivery. And while home care aides are not mere puppets of the industry—they are also agents in thwarting and acting out these practices—the result has largely been the failure to develop worker-based strategies.

### Do We Need Home Care Agencies?

This leads one to wonder: If home care agencies have been sites of exploitation and isolation for workers, should we eliminate those agencies and organize home care services differently? Consider, for example, the move in some states to independent provider programs or consumer-driven service models. According to these approaches, home care "consumers" directly control delivery of their home care services. Rather than going through a home care agency, for example, individuals are given the financial means to hire the caretaker of their choice. This means that individuals in need of care may use their government funding to hire family members and that they have direct control over the hiring, firing, scheduling, supervision, and payment of home care workers.

Given its emphasis on consumer choice and satisfaction, this model has been supported by many persons in the disabled community. Persons with disabilities who have had the opportunity to oversee and take charge of their own care services feel a sense of empowerment when they control the conditions under which they receive assistance. Instead of being the passive recipients of care, and thus rendered helpless and dependent on the care of others, independent provider programs and consumer-driver service models encourage disabled persons to be active agents in securing and overseeing their own care. Anita Silvers claims:

> Modeling social organization on being cared for and caring thus appears to make compliant behavior a mandate for persons with disabilities. For them, submissiveness remains the price of good treatment. In a framework of moral relations in which some must make themselves vulnerable so that others can be worthy of their trust —that is, in paternalistic systems, in which those viewed as incompetent are coerced into compliance "for their own good"—people with disabilities are typecast as subordinate. (100)

Insofar as these new models thwart typecasting of disabled persons as subordinates, they are desirable ways of organizing care services. And given my concern with the way home care agencies are organized, the elimination of this level of bureaucracy may seem justified. Indeed, I applaud the move toward client-controlled strategies, where those in need of care are no longer at the mercy of providers that require their compliance in order to receive it. But I am not convinced that such a move in itself empowers either caretakers or care recipients.

We need a different, more radical, strategy for securing respect and rights for care recipients and working conditions for caretakers, a strategy that involves coalition building. As long as home care workers face terrible wages, uneven work hours, lack of benefits (including health care insurance, sick pay, and paid vacation), and unskilled status, clients will continue to experience hardship in finding good care workers. Placing small care stipends in the hands of clients themselves will not solve these problems. On the contrary, workers will continue to move in and out of the home care industry, and recruitment and retention problems will only be passed along to clients. Persons in need of assistance will have to put up with continued substandard care.

For example, the results of an Access Living focus group on personal assistants (conducted by Loyola University's Center for Urban Research and Learning)[3] indicated the persistence of serious care problems. One client voiced the following worries and complaints: "People didn't know what to do. They were unqualified, on drugs. I had to tell them everything to do. They were very temperamental or wouldn't come into work. There was some theft. I got a list of seven people from Access Living. I called everyone and got no response." Another person who organized her own care voiced similar problems, claiming, "I had the same situations. I got a PA (personal attendant) from Intrim and had some of the same issues, like taking things. They should give a drug test. It's a low-skill job and underpaid, and they'll just send us anybody. They turn out to be drug addicts and alcoholics. You have to find someone from your church or in your family."

When asked why they experienced such difficulties, focus group participants indicated that economic and social problems persist. For example, one person said, "It's money, too. It's hard for anyone to live off of $5.56 an hour. You're not paying the guy nothing, he's not gonna take good care of you." Another claimed, "It's because they don't screen people. It's a low-paying job, and you get people who didn't go past the third or fourth grade. It's underpaid, so they figure they can do anything they want to us."

While eliminating home care agencies may seem like the solution to many home care ills, it is not clear that consumer-directed care will eliminate or even reduce the serious problems currently bound up with home care. Allowing clients to directly pay for and oversee their home care provision only seems to transfer macro problems to the micro level of the individual client's home.

A better approach, then, would incorporate the caretakers' needs and perspectives into the mode of care delivery. The problem with independent provider programs and consumer-driven service models is that they are not concerned with the "big picture" in home care. These programs may prove desirable for the same reasons home care rose in popularity: because it is cheaper for states to let individuals hire their own caretakers than to oversee it on the state level. For example, studies indicate that independent provider arrangements are cheaper than a home care agency–based approach because labor and administrative costs are lowered.[4] These new programs avoid the overhead associated with hiring, training, and supervising workers and with agency monitoring of home care contracts. As some home care theorists have indicated, independent provider programs are used by states to move the sickest or most disabled clients into this sector in order to minimize program costs. The result is that the most vulnerable clients—those requiring more involved care—may be served by untrained and unsupervised workers (Feldman et al.).

I object to independent provider programs and consumer-driven service models, then, because they once again represent a shifting of state responsibility to the individual. The language of choice and autonomy may be appealing, but these models of providing care actually fail in these respects. While some persons with disabilities have had success in securing caretakers who are trained and reliable, many others are left frustrated and angry.

Furthermore, these clients are not really empowered when they are at the mercy of individual caretakers who may not show up for work, who may steal from them, who may take drugs or drink on the job, and who are likely to leave the industry within a short period of time. The state should not use these programs as a way of deflecting responsibility for the care of its citizens.

### Taking Care of Business

When I claim that we require coalition-building strategies, I refer to those approaches that reject the pitting of client against caretaker and that refuse to allow the government to transfer caretaking responsibility to private citizens. As I suggested in chapter 5, while affirmative reform strategies like paid family caretaking may be necessary in the short run, we need a longer view of our home care goals. Shifting responsibility from the state to individual clients by giving clients a small sum with which to purchase their care services should not be the long-term answer. Indeed, such a move is not an ethically sound long-term strategy, as our experiments thus far with home care have taught us.[5] Giving citizens with care needs small stipends with which to hire caretakers will not ensure that either party will flourish; rather, both will suffer the effects of extremely low pay, overwork, and an unstable workforce. Furthermore, a move toward independent providers doesn't even scratch the surface of the Marxist concerns for alienation, meaningful labor, and value that I previously mentioned. Something more is required.

The "more" to which I am referring is a move toward democratizing home care, and the chief way to achieve such democratization is through unionizing home care workers. Indeed, that such workers are starting to take control over their work lives is evidenced by the slow move toward trade unions. For example, in 1999 the Service Employees International Union (SEIU) gained a major foothold in the rapidly expanding labor pool of people who do home care work by adding 75,000 home health care workers to their membership.[6] Workers in California organized to ensure fair wages, work hours, and benefits and to lower home care industry turnover rates, which are notoriously high. These worker demands echo calls that other home care theorists have made to democratize home care. As Rebecca Donovan argued over a decade ago,

> The system of employment must be based on a philosophy which views the paraprofessional home care worker as a valued member of the health care team with active involvement in planning patient care. Their em-

ployment must be structured accordingly. The core workforce should be salaried employees with guaranteed work hours that include training, supervision, and record-keeping. Salaries and fringe benefits should be comparable to similar employment in health care institutions . . . with sick leave, vacation time, comprehensive health benefits, and retirement plans. In addition, career ladders should be established with opportunities for promotion and advancement within the industry. (113)

More recently, too, we are seeing the genesis of home care agencies that are worker owned and operated. For example, Cooperative Home Care Associates in the South Bronx offers a program by which workers receive a better hourly wage as well as health benefits, life insurance, a stake in the company, and—for the best workers—a chance of being promoted into management. This approach refuses to view and treat home care aides as "bedpan dumpers" and rather invests in the workers themselves. As one report indicates, by investing in its workforce, "Cooperative has done what few agencies have managed: retained experienced, dedicated workers. Staff turnover is less than 20 percent per year, half the industry average."[7] Companies like Cooperative—which are being replicated in other cities in the United States—are attempting to create a democratic workplace that ultimately benefits everyone.

In short, the coalition-building for which I am arguing is not found solely in labor unions but may be achieved in various ways. While I approve heartily of the organizing efforts of home care workers who have joined the SEIU within the past decade, I do not think that this is the only way to ensure justice for caretakers (and, by extension, care recipients) in home care. Moves toward worker-owned and -operated companies may also have the desired democratizing effect.[8] In his recent work, Milton Fisk treats the issue of trade unions and argues that the "labor politics thesis"— that health care can only be transformed through trade unions or a labor party—is flawed. As he indicates, histories in Canada, the United States, and Mexico indicate that gains were won without being led by trade unions. He argues that we need to develop a new class politics that comes not from one point of struggle but from several. While not all groups that come together will share all concerns, Fisk asserts that they will find common cause in organizing around health care reform (193).

As I see it, union organizing and worker-owned and -operated agencies are the surest ways to achieve the goals for which I have been arguing in this book. Like Fisk, I see the "new class politics" as going beyond workers' class-based concerns to include other strands in the struggle against oppression. Here I would include concerns for race (given that home care workers are largely minorities), gender (since most employees are women), and age (since most home care clients are elderly). By moving health care out of the for-profit sector, we move home health care, too. This avoids waiting for change in the social value of care work—a change that I am highly skeptical will ever occur on its own—and properly recognizes the state's role in seeing to the good care of its citizens. Thus, I envision changes that are effected both at the state level and by grassroots movements initiated by workers themselves.

But this is only part of the puzzle. The other part, for which I have been arguing throughout this book, is a feminist-based critique of home care that places women at the fore. Since I have already rehearsed the reasons for seeing home health care as an explicitly feminist issue, in what follows I will pursue the critique that a standard of care must be put in place before we appeal to cost-based concerns. By inverting the equation so that we allow economic considerations to determine what care we can afford, we continue to allow the state to free-ride on women's care work.

### Righting Wrongs: Putting Care First

> If we set up an economy in which "nice guys and gals finish last," we end up with an economy in which nice guys and gals are exploited to extinction. Our economic system tends to waste natural human capabilities for care and love in much the same way that we waste free goods like air and water. Therefore, we can't continue simply to rely on the "natural" provision of care—we need to engage in specific forms of collective action aimed to protect, enhance, and expand it. (Folbre and Ferguson, 98)

The final challenge in making my feminist case for the revision of home care involves arguing for political and economic justice for female caretakers without reducing care to something that can be easily priced. In what follows, I will argue that the caretaking offered by women in the United States is often done at their own peril or at peril to their families—ironically, the very persons that their care work is meant to protect! These perils take the form of little to no income for their work, physical exhaustion, emotional and psychological distress, working a "double day," and being stretched to the breaking point on time commitments. Such conditions are not at all conducive to flourishing families (again, something that care work is meant to produce). To offset the likelihood of these dangers, we need to give caretakers decent pay and/or benefits, so that the kind of "natural" familial care of which Joan Tronto and Nel Noddings write so approvingly can be supported. But this does not mean that care can or should be reduced to a market value that costs out the mechanics behind caretaking.

Moral caring goes beyond the physical tasks of caring for persons; for this reason, I appeal to a feminist ethic of care to ground caring practices. An ethic of care centralizes practices of caring for and about persons, so that nurturing, love, respect, interdependence, and responsiveness are given pride of place. But as chapter 3 indicates, the care ethic that we invoke must be a public one that places women's care in its proper social, political, and economic context. So any appeal to a care ethic should not obscure political concerns for women's fair and equal treatment.

Ultimately, we must begin with the notions of "public" and "private" life of which I was critical in chapter 1. As I argued, the notion of public life is historically associated with the masculine; the notion of private life, with the feminine. And while individuals may be starting to question the meaning and usefulness of this distinction, no practice presses it more than home health care. Indeed, one could see home care as a test case for the public/private distinction, for the practice blurs the boundaries between the two spheres. Though I have referred to notions of public and private life throughout this book, I have done so self-consciously, for, especially in the arena of home care, the distinctions between the two spheres are becoming increasingly fuzzy. Yes, home care takes place within the "privacy" of individuals' homes, where individual preferences reign supreme. But this does not mean that home care aides enter a domain that is free of social and political meanings. On the contrary, what goes on in that "private" space both affects and is affected by the so-called public domain.

So I begin with the broadest question, which concerns how to challenge the present ideological split between public and private spheres of life. Feminists have puzzled over this for some time. And while the project of challenging this ideology may seem daunting, indeed, I assert that we express a deep suspicion of this division in our everyday practices. In theory, our public lives are distinct from our private ones; in practice, the line between the two is much less clear. Caring is the perfect example of this fuzziness, for while it is understood as a private relationship between private individuals, it is at the same time called upon by the state in the support and protection of vulnerable citizens. Thus, even something as private as caring is a public act.

Furthermore, the distinction between public and private spheres is *itself* determined in the public sphere. There is no a priori distinction between these two domains; rather, what counts as private or public concerns is set out in politics, law, and public policy. These concerns are thus humanly, not divinely (or naturally) created. The spheres of public and private life are relativized such that they are open to contestation and change.[9] This is important to my ultimate argument that care should be viewed and treated as a public good on par with those of clean air, potable water, and other recognized common goods.

If what counts as "public" or "private" is alterable, then we have grounds for rethinking the offhand rejection of caretaking as a public good. By simply appealing to tradition or history, we fail to offer any solid justification for continuing to treat care as a private endeavor. Rather, if we consider feminist strategies for re-visioning caretaking, we begin to appreciate the radical claim that care work *is* work and, moreover, that it is work of public (not just private) value. As Eva Kittay claims,

> If dependency is not part of one's daily life, it is easy and convenient to ignore it. After all, what does cleaning bedpans or comforting a teary toddler have to do with matters of State, matters of finance, or the world of culture? The answer, of course, is *everything*. Yet our own dependency and the dependency of others has been conveniently kept out-of-sight, tucked away metaphorically and literally, attended to by women who have only aspired to and have not yet achieved full citizenship. (1999, 184)

In order to take care seriously as a public good, then, we need to demonstrate that it is something in which most Americans have an interest. To do this, we need to show that public care provision (which would involve the state at a basic level) is a better plan than leaving caretaking and the fulfillment of care needs to individuals within private relationships. And to make this argument, we need to further show that public care promotes the kinds of human flourishing, function, and capabilities that are an important part of our common public life. For example, I would need to show that the fulfillment of my Aunt Sally's care needs go well beyond her own ability to function, to include the common good of respect for individuals in our communities. Beyond this, a function or capabilities approach points us to such important goods as the importance of freedom, democracy (in terms of the fair and inclusive discourse I highlighted in chapter 5), and autonomy.

But why autonomy? Given what I have argued in previous chapters, it may seem incongruous to claim that a capabilities approach helps to protect autonomy, especially if human relationships are marked by relationality and dependency. Yet the feminist conception of relational autonomy that I have put forth rejects the ascription of civic privileges to only those capable of functioning independently of others' care. Since we are all in relationships of caretaking or receiving (and sometimes both at the same time), autonomy should not be taken to imply an independent, isolated agent who is unencumbered by his own care needs or by the care demands of others. In the sense I am proposing, autonomy is socially desirable and a basic goal that should be fostered. But autonomy is not an intrinsic good; rather, it is instrumental to an individual's ability to secure her own conception of the good. On this understanding, autonomy is not a necessary condition for political participation but an instrumental good that should be fostered in each citizen insofar as each is able to develop it.[10] Rather than presuming equal capacity on the part of each citizen, then, my conception of autonomy recognizes that citizens start with different functional positions with regard to abilities and potential. As Kittay points out, her severely disabled daughter may not ever resemble the autonomous, free, fully functioning agent that is so characteristic of political life. But, as she puts it, "Perhaps what her case really tells us is, first that it is not productivity and independence that matter, but the full flourishing of each member of the community, and, second, that a fully flourishing life involves family, community, and the interdependence of those with whom we share family and community" (2000, 73).

So autonomy is achieved through a citizenry's collective enablement of possibilities and capacities. This conception recognizes that the general drive toward self-sufficiency is not innately given but is learned, and that one's success or failure in achieving it is related to the social context within which one is living. Still, that autonomy has this social component does not mean that we should minimize an individual's ability to choose her own ends. It should still matter to us that individuals come up with their own conception of how they want to live their lives, that they are agents' own conceptions, and that they directly relate to individuals' capacity to flourish. To understand autonomy in this way is to understand it as the ability to convert goods and resources into functionings, or what Amartya Sen calls "capabilities."

Sen's capabilities approach leads us to question the way that primary goods (like the means to fulfill care needs) are differently countenanced by individuals. Suppose, returning to independent provider programs for a moment, that clients are given equal monies with which to purchase home care services from a pool of available workers. In this scenario, two clients are offered the same means to secure care services, but one client requires minimal services, like help with her grocery shopping and housekeeping, while another client requires more intensive care involving transfers from bed to wheelchair, help with bathing and dressing, catheter care, and so on. Since client A's needs are less demanding, she is far more likely to find workers who will assist her for the available monies; but client B's more intensive care needs make it far less likely that she will find a caretaker who will do the work for the going rate. Put simply, because client B is differently positioned, she has difficulty in converting the available funding into a substantive conception of her own good. The money given to both clients may represent our social assurance of the same primary goods for citizens, but it doesn't result in the expression of equal capabilities. As this example shows, even an equitable distribution of primary goods (like financial resources) may result in an extensive lack of opportunity in citizens' pursuit of their substantive ends. With his capabilities approach, Sen leads us to consider not just what primary goods are universally available but what mechanisms are in place for converting those goods into individual human flourishing. Client B cannot express her capabilities, or flourish, if she doesn't have the structures in place that enable her to pursue her job outside of her home— that is, if she can't get out of her home because there is no one willing to come for $5.50 per hour and assist her with her intensive care needs.

In a similar way, as feminists are arguing, dependents and care workers are socially positioned such that they are rendered incapable of achieving the ends they set for themselves. For example, as Kittay argues, in the case of persons with totalizing dependencies (individuals with severe mental disabilities, for example), the deeply dependent person must rely on the caretaker to achieve the dependent's well-being and to fulfill her substantive conception of the good.[11] At a foundational level, caretakers need social structures and supports in place (such as financial support, educational support, respite care services) in order to attend to the specific needs of the charge. The caretaker, then, must be given support in converting the initial set of goods into the substantive means of achieving the dependent person's ends.

Beyond this support, however, caretakers must be given the opportunity to meet their own conceptions of the good, too. This is not to say that a society must necessarily spend huge amounts of money to fulfill caretakers' conceptions of the good, but just that caretakers should not unfairly and unequally experience impediments to their realization. And these impediments should not be understood as arising on the individual level. On the contrary, as Kittay argues, "When dependency work is done by a specifiable social group, the vulnerability of the dependency worker will be a function not only of her individual situation, but also of the status of her social group" (1999, 46). This means that caretakers as a group should not face impediments to their capabilities that other "care-free" citizens do not face. Furthermore, as Kittay points out, since good caretakers express the moral quality of being transparent selves—that is, the caretaker's self must be transparent to the needs of the cared-for if good care is to take place—the caretakers are again atypically positioned such that they are not simply the disinterested or self-interested self that liberal theory demands. Rather, caretakers are "passionately interested" selves, with their interest "vested in the well-being of another" (1999, 53).

Given the caretaker's investment in her charge, we need to be sensitive to the impact this personal investment is likely to have on her ability to meet her own needs. As I indicated in chapter 3, Kittay rightly advocates a conception of "doulia"—nested dependencies—whereby the caretaker's needs are attended to by others who are involved in the web of care. But on Kittay's model, one must be involved in caretaking in order to invoke the doulia principle. So her model may ultimately prove problematic in that it doesn't require broader social questioning of who does the care work in our society (and who escapes it). All her principle of doulia may require is that we ensure caretakers have support in their caring enterprises and that caretakers are cared for. What this does not do, however, is ensure that caretakers are provided with the means for the pursuit of their own conceptions of the good. If Kittay's proposal is to align well with Sen's capabilities model, then, she should provide means by which caretakers are freed from responsibility for attending to charges' needs so that they can pursue their own. Beyond providing welfare provisions, the caretaker should have agent maneuverability to develop her own interests as she sees fit.

The importance of developing capabilities, especially where it is largely women who are denied this opportunity, is apparent in the home care arena. As I have indicated, it is women (both paid and unpaid) who largely surrender their own goals, plans, and career paths in order to care for citizens in need of care. Women who take up paid home care service, for example, become so bogged down in the care needs of others, and are so busy doing enough care work to put food on the table, that their opportunities to develop their own substantive conceptions of the good are lost. Many home care workers cite other life plans—to return to school, to take nursing classes, to learn business administration so they can move up or out of the home care industry—yet these plans often fall by the wayside, as workers lack an enabling society that supports the development of other capabilities while they are performing care work.

While dependency may be a settled fact, arrangements concerning the care of dependents are not. It just so happens that, historically, women have done the lion's share of caretaking in this culture. But this says much more about social arrangements than it does about any connection between women and caring. Despite the naturalizing of women's care work, it is an historically contingent fact that women are caretakers and that caring is linked to the private realm of the home and family. And just as I am arguing that we should revise our notions of caretaking as part of the "private" realm, so I am arguing that we should revise our notion of caretaking as a feminine practice and virtue.

*Rethinking the Need for a Standard of Care*

Alasdair MacIntyre takes a critical view of the way in which care-taking resources are distributed in the United States. According to him, a kind of mean-spirited economic scheme has determined what kind of care our society will provide for citizens. In short, MacIntyre argues that a moral reversal has taken place, where economic considerations have determined what kind of care we can afford, rather than having citizens collectively determine what kind of care we want and then determining how to provide it. As he claims,

> We should not begin by asking what resources we now provide for the care of the mentally retarded and the mentally ill and then allow the present scale and organization of those resources to set limits to the care that we provide in particular cases. We need instead to begin from a justified standard of care, so that we can ask how, in the light of that standard, our overall resources ought to be allocated. Our budget-making should be informed by our standards and not vice-versa. Of course it would be imprudent and therefore quite wrong for a society to risk the danger of bankruptcy by unwise and excessive allocations for this or any other purpose. But the way to avoid that risk without surrendering to the often mean-spirited allocations of the status quo is for the members of a society to think through together how their shared resources ought to be allocated in light of their various responsibilities. And some of those responsibilities cannot be defined without a standard of care. (82)

But, as MacIntyre claims, the standard of care must not be defined by current practice or by professionals. The way care is currently meted out does not tell us what standard of care we ought to have. Moreover, MacIntyre rejects the setting of care standards by professionals, like physicians and policymakers. By allowing an elite group of individuals to set the standard of care to which all citizens will be held, we are failing to see such standard-setting as a democratic, community process. Determining how we ought to care for citizens, and what level of care is morally decent, he argues, should be done democratically, by all of us. Furthermore, a standard of care must be set in light of the care virtues that make for the common good of all who live in a society of mutual dependence and mutual caring.

MacIntyre argues that appeals to duty or obligation only lead to a grudging, minimalist ethic. A truly virtuous society will understand that care for self is tied to community. That individuals flourish and that capacities are fulfilled when care is taken as a public, common good is, on his account, what makes care a virtue. MacIntyre's virtues approach, then, fits well with Sen's account of capabilities, where receiving and learning how to give loving care are valuable both for their own sake and for the other capabilities that such care supports.

Furthermore, MacIntyre argues that, in order to ever pay caretakers fairly, we need to change. A standard of care should include consideration for the individuals and ideals to which we are committed. By considering these factors, he claims, we can sketch out what is "defective" in persons who fail to uphold an adequate standard of care. As MacIntyre puts it, citizens defective in the moral virtue of care will "not take the possibility of their or their children pursuing a career as a provider of care for the disabled as having any great claim upon them or theirs and they will not understand the importance of raising the wages paid to and enhancing the status and prestige enjoyed by those who give their lives to such caregiving" (85). MacIntyre asserts that we can't put resources toward protecting agency until we know what it is we are to protect. He first asks, What is the standard of care we want in place?

While I strongly support MacIntyre's communitarian/virtues approach, I argue that his position should be strengthened by adopting a strong feminist dimension. While he roots care in communities and sees virtue as attached to care, he does not see that virtues are not universally applied to all citizens. Some virtues, for example, are feminized; in this case, care is a particularly "feminine" virtue. Caretaking for the vulnerable and dependent in our society isn't a general community problem, then, but a problem for women in particular. Feminists have been highly critical of discourses that overlook the political implications of care as a feminine virtue. In MacIntyre's case, by failing to include these considerations, he fails to see why a standard of care appears chimerical. On a feminist account of care and virtue, we set a lowball standard of care because the feminine care expectations are already set in place. In other words, we have failed to meet the need for a standard of care because there has been no need to set one. Our private, feminized system of care has long been in place to deal with caretaking needs.

Nevertheless, MacIntyre's point is well worth noting here. We have embarked on the home health care enterprise absent any clear community perspective on what we hope to gain. Because of this lack of common vision, home care practices have been governed by a minimalist ethic that focuses on cutting costs and limiting care. In much the same way, MacIntyre is arguing, we have engaged in policymaking surrounding people with disabilities absent any clear sense of what standard of care we want in place for them.[12]

## Practical Identities as a Primary Good

MacIntyre's call for a standard of care is helpful in thinking through what is wrong with current home care practice. As he suggests, at least part of the problem is that we practice care absent any collective, community determination of what standard should be in place. But MacIntyre's position lacks the depth that a feminist critique adds to considerations of care and community standards. And he doesn't address the way that identities are bound up with caretaking such that citizens' very selves—and not just their social status as contributing members of society—are at risk.

James Lindemann Nelson has also addressed the problem of determining a reasonable standard of care. Yet Nelson focuses not only on care as a virtue and a public good. He also considers ontological issues in caretaking. In brief, he claims that the shift of health care responsibilities to families raises important questions about our very selves or, as Christine Korsgaard puts it, our "practical identities." Nelson quotes Korsgaard's definition of a practical identity as "a description under which you find your life to be worth living and your actions to be worth undertaking." According to Nelson, the "wrongs" of health care systems are perpetrated where the identities that form who we are, that make "central contributions to our overall sense of self," are wrenched from us.

> Reflecting on the importance of practical identities is on point because the kind of intensive caregiving increasingly demanded of families is not merely a matter of shifting resources from one area of an organization's endeavors to another. Rather, it is very likely to involve a restructuring of people's most basic projects—those activities that are deeply implicated in some of the most fundamental and personally significant ways that people identify themselves. One's ability to take on and maintain an identity as, say, a breadwinner, a professional, a student, or even a spouse, may be impaired or blocked. (In press)

While Nelson acknowledges the need to change the material conditions under which families (and, I would add, paid caretakers) give care, he points to deeper problems by which intensive caretaking demands result in the destruction of practical identities. This, he claims, is where the deep injustice of current care practices are to be found. For just as we view health care as a primary good—as key to our pursuit of our own specific visions of the good—so, too, is the maintenance of our practical identities. Health, according to bioethicist Norman Daniels, allows for the maintenance of a "normal opportunity range."[13] Yet Nelson claims that this is equally true of the formation and maintenance of practical identities. He thus ties the formation of this identity to normal (human) species functioning and asserts that the ability to do this is "intimately caught up with our opportunity range" (in press).

This brings Nelson back to my previous discussion of Sen's capabilities model. Insofar as Nelson links the formation and maintenance of our practical identities with a normal opportunity range, and insofar as he sees these identities are part of normal species functioning, they are linked to the development of human capabilities. Without this kind of fundamental identity around which to formulate a life plan, one is not enabled in the development of one's capabilities; human flourishing is stunted or denied, and individuals may become, as Ann Ferguson puts it, "sociopathic . . . and hence a public cost" (Folbre and Ferguson, 102). In a real sense, then, these practical identities are both personal and public goods, and where human agency blocks or erodes the formation and maintenance of them, a moral wrong is committed.

It is neither necessary nor inevitable that care work results in the fracturing or fragmentation of practical identities; rather, such effects are the result of a badly constructed system of care. For example, one of my identities may be as the loving daughter of an elderly parent. Yet insofar as my parent's care demands fall upon me and me alone, I may find it impossible to maintain that identity. Rather than being the loving, supportive daughter with which I deeply identify, the caretaking pressures may render me a harsh, irritable, physically or verbally abusive caretaker who bristles with each need expressed by my elderly parent. According to Nelson's account, then, the wrongs are expressed not just in my abusive treatment of my elderly parent but in the fracturing of my identity. Until we appreciate the extent to which current home care practices fragment our practical identities, we will lack a deep appreciation for the moral problems with home health care.

By bringing together the theoretically rich feminist and Marxist approaches and applying them to the home care enterprise, we better understand what is needed to render home care practice ethical. I argue that, in isolation, neither a feminist nor a Marxist approach will do. Rather, we need a combination of the two to identify processes of alienation and self-fragmentation and gender-based ascriptions of care work that leave women shouldering the caretaking burden in most western cultures. By invoking these critical perspectives, we can develop a better, less exploitative, and more inclusive framework for the practice of home health care.

## Conclusion

This chapter has considered the question of whether home care can be reformed. Chapters 1 through 5 indicate the many problems that are bound up with current home care practice; this chapter considers ways of addressing those problems. As I have argued, while certain short-term strategies may be justified to render home care as minimally exploitative as possible (for example, by paying family caretakers), we need a longer view of the ethics of home care. At the very least, home care should not be run on a for-profit basis: As long as it is modeled on the managed care system of health care, it stands little chance of being reformed. In addition, home care must be democratized by ensuring that even the "lowliest" of home care workers have some control over their working conditions. This democratization can be achieved through a variety of means, including unionizing and developing worker owned and operated agencies, where aides have meaningful input into their work.

With regard to democratizing home care, we also need to develop a standard of care—a call most recently and forcefully made by MacIntyre. Without such a standard in place we will continue to treat caretaking in a miserly and penurious fashion; we will also lack the necessary community support for good caretaking practice. And as MacIntyre indicates, from a good, supportive, democratic community comes a decent standard of care. Until communities develop such standards, they will continue to develop care policies absent any real sense of what is a morally decent level of care provision.

Finally, as Nelson so clearly articulates, basic issues of personal identity are bound up with ethical questions concerning home health care. Poor support for caretaking results in fragmented identities, or it may at the very least require that caretakers restructure their most basic life projects to accommodate dependents' care needs. And while some caretakers may choose to make accommodations in their lifestyles and their identities in order to provide the necessary care, others do not so choose. In such cases, care work is foisted on individuals in ways that are destructive of their very identities, and this can result in an unhappy situation for both caretakers and cared-for. As such identity concerns illustrate, the deep injustice of current care practices extend beyond economic and physical exploitation.

Nelson's critique fits nicely with Sen's model, which allows us to consider society's responsibility for developing caretakers' capabilities. Sen leads us to consider the importance of developing individuals' functioning or capabilities beyond caretaking, such that they are supported in developing their own substantive conceptions of the good. Currently, the mostly female care workforce is so burdened with the care needs of others that their opportunities to develop their conceptions of the good (and, by extension, their identities) are lost. The other plans that make caretakers' lives meaningful—returning to school, learning business administration, and so on—fall by the wayside, resulting in a lack of opportunity to develop other capabilities while they are performing care work. Ultimately this means that when their caretaking years are over, they are unprepared and incapable of doing other kinds of meaningful work.[14] A robust account of the ethics of home care, then, must consider its impact on the development and sustaining of practical identities and the ways that capabilities remain undeveloped because of intensive care demands.

These considerations would be pressing enough without adding demographic pressures. As many scholars have indicated, we are heading toward an aging society, where soon citizens over age 65 will outnumber citizens who are participating in the workforce. Some predict that by 2010, the Medicare system that finances care for the elderly will experience a serious crisis.[15]

Indeed, as Philip Brickner has claimed,

> A rapid and substantial increase in the numbers of older individuals in our country is taking place. The number of persons in the United States aged 85 years old or more grew by 232% in the past 3 decades. In contrast, the numbers of those 65 and older grew by 89% and the total population by only 39%. . . . Projections are that the 12% of the population now 65 and older will double in percentage by the year 2020. Those 85 and over are expected to quadruple in percentage. (45)

Given these demographics, the call to reform home care will become ever more urgent as our population ages.

The greatest challenge that we will face in the next few decades will involve providing the best care possible for a growing population of elderly citizens. Since home-based care is the current paradigm, and people are likely to continue to treasure their homes over institutional sites, we must negotiate the needs of dependent citizens to receive at-home care and the needs of caretakers to receive both decent pay and recognition for the value of their work. Failure to take these challenges seriously could have tragic results. Indeed, as Mark Waymack has noted,

> If we understand how the activity of sensitive, humane home care workers can be crucial for maintaining the moral sense of self, the sense of integrity, the very self-identity of their clients, then we can easily see the

deep moral importance of their work. Without such support, the frail face the impossible choice. Borrowing from and slightly altering the words of Samuel Beckett ["It is suicide to be abroad. But what is it to be at home, Mr. Tyler, what is it to be at home? A lingering dissolution"] . . . it would be suicide to be institutionalized, but to remain at home without assistance would be a lingering dissolution. (59)

# NOTES

## Introduction

1. Indeed, the problem remains of how—and when—to accomplish ethics training in home care, given the impossibility of finding a common meeting time for aides and given the wide variety of the health care aides' backgrounds and experience.

2. This also explains why aides are matched with cases that are far beyond their caretaking capacity. Supervisors become so desperate for an aide that they will assign unqualified workers to clients with skilled care needs.

3. Indeed, one aptly entitled article, "Women's Sense of Responsibility for the Care of Old People: 'But Who Else Is Going to Do It?'" deals with this very issue of women's sense of responsibility for caretaking. See Aronson (1992).

4. "Community-based" care means care that is accomplished outside of institutions, within the broader community. Home care is one type of community-based care, since it supposedly takes place within the community, is overseen by the community-at-large, and is more inclusive of the cared-for. Yet Eva Kittay challenges the assumption that community-based care provides *better* care by asking, "Might not a well-run institution with a devoted administrative staff that guarantees a uniform level of good-quality care be preferable even to a small group home in which the quality of care can be more directly subject to the vicissitudes of personnel (whose turnover rates are high) and inadequate?" (2000, 71).

5. "Caring for Ailing Aged Linked to Strain, Death," *Chicago Tribune,* December 15, 1999.

6. While a client's specific request for a female caretaker does make an issue of sex and gender, it is not an instance of *sexism*. It is not on irrelevant grounds, for example, that an elderly women specifies a female caretaker when she requires assistance with bathing and peri (or genital) care. Elderly women may justifiably prefer female caretakers to perform such intimate tasks.

7. Autonomous people, according to the Kantian tradition, are self-governing, have reason and will, and have the capacity to make their own choices and develop their own life plans. Traditionally, autonomy requires respect for individual persons, meaning one person does not have authority over another and thus should not coerce others, limit their activities, or impose his will on others. Privacy rights—and rights to noninterference—are directly associated with this principle of autonomy. As I will argue later in this book, the conception of autonomy as privacy or noninterference is not helpful to an ethical analysis of home health care.

8. Thanks to my colleague David Ozar for helping me think through this issue of autonomy in long-term care situations.

9. Martha Holstein (1999, 2001), Joan Tronto (1993, 1998), and Rosalie Kane and Carrie Levin (1998) have offered feminist ethical treatments of home health care.

## 1. Why Home Care?

1. My vision on this issue has been trained by thinkers like Martha Fineman, Eva Kittay, Susan Moller Okin, and Catharine MacKinnon. These feminists have begun to lay the groundwork for a feminist theory of the state (as MacKinnon calls it), one which includes attention to remuneration for women's caretaking in liberal democratic, capitalist societies. See Fineman's argument (2000) for the formal recognition of women's caretaking that results in a huge subsidy to the state.

2. More recently, studies indicate that home health care is *not* less expensive than institution-based care. While there have certainly been savings in the areas of hospital and nursing home care, the increasing technologization of home care services and the increasing number of patients requiring them means that savings may not be as great as predicted. See Arno, Levine, and Memmott (1999).

3. This widespread lack of insurance results from unemployment (since many Americans are either unemployed or are only employed part-time) and employment with companies that are too small to provide health care benefits to employees. An employer-based health insurance system means that only large companies with a huge employee base can afford to insure employees through a system of managed care. In addition, Medicaid is only available to citizens who are devastatingly poor, meaning that many Americans, while gainfully employed, do not have any health insurance whatsoever.

4. According to Feder, Komisar, and Niefeld, "In 1998 Medicaid financed about 40 percent of the nation's long-term care spending of $150 billion and 44 percent of spending on nursing home care" (2000, 41).

5. Ginger Orr, "Home-Care Agencies Seek Funding Remedy," *Chicago Tribune,* May 2, 2000.

6. "Caring for Ailing Aged Linked to Strain, Death," *Chicago Tribune,* December 15, 1999.

7. For examples of feminist critiques of familial caretaking, see Tronto (1998) and Noddings (1996); for sociological accounts, see Finch and Groves (1983); for legal treatments, see Minow (1990); and for bioethical critiques, see Nelson (2002).

8. Other examples include Dalley (1984), Aronson (1992), and Kittay (1999).

9. For good accounts of the acute care paradigm, see Hinton-Walker (1993), Moros et al. (1991), and Roth and Harrison (1991).

10. While I am critical of traditional conceptions of autonomy, I will later argue that a feminist conception of relational autonomy addresses the reality of human relationships. Such a relational conception might get us beyond the acute care paradigm that reigns supreme in health care.

11. Notice this isolates and medicalizes individuals, rendering their social situations and their relationships as *impediments* to their autonomy. Chapter 4 will argue that this model wrongly characterizes human beings, failing to account for the ways in which our autonomy is socially constituted and upheld.

12. Simone de Beauvoir (1980) criticizes the repetitive, "nonproductive" nature of women's work. She uses the example of housework and cooking, where the tasks are endless and repetitive. Women are still considered "nonproductive" in our society despite our staggering numbers on the job market in both full-time and part-time jobs.

13. For a full account of this caretaking relationship, see "Blacks Carry Load of Care for Their Elderly," *New York Times,* March 15, 1998.

14. "Blacks Carry Load."

15. "Blacks Carry Load."

16. "Blacks Carry Load."

17. Here I have in mind the lowest paid sector of home care workers: home care aides, those who do the unskilled work of helping clients complete their ADLs and IADLs. While there is also a paucity of *skilled* home care professionals, my focus in this book is on the lower skill levels, where caretakers are most exploited by the home care system.

18. See Donovan (1989) and Feldman (1997).

19. For an excellent account of the exploitation of migrant workers, see Ingram (2000). As he points out, migrant and other immigrant workers are paid wages lower than is allowable for American citizens.

20. See Feldman (1997).

### 2. Examining Philosophies of Home Care

1. I take this notion of "central values" from Ozar and Sokol (1994).

2. For an excellent discussion of the distinction between caring for and caring about, see Joan Tronto (1998).

3. Note that such breadth is unique to the practice of home health care. Medical professions are usually understood as practices with distinct bodies of knowledge and specific training, so anesthesiologists, psychiatrists, podiatrists, and pediatricians are skilled experts in particular areas of medicine. I argue that home health care's low status is connected to the nonspecific nature of its practice and its perceived lack of a body of knowledge common to other health care professions.

4. For a nice discussion of the distinction between professional and nonprofessional work, see Kittay (1999, 38–41).

5. Home care aides live out the tension, then, between their obligation to their employer (their commitment to corporate values) and their obligation to their clients (kinlike obligations). They walk a fine line between the two and are often left in unhappy situations.

6. Note, however, that in situations of home care, reciprocity can be strained. Care recipients are sometimes incapable of returning care or of recognizing their caretakers as concrete others. In such cases, the formal conception of reciprocity proves even more unsatisfactory. For an excellent account of this problem of reciprocity, see Kittay (1999).

7. At my home care agency, once clients were no longer capable of taking their own medication, they were shifted from home to institution. There was a sometimes spurious distinction between clients "taking their own medication" and having someone else administer it: aides were allowed to hold the client's hand to steady it

and even raise the client's hand to her mouth, but we were not allowed to simply deliver the medications by our own hands. Aides regularly broke this rule and would chart a client's ability to self-medicate, in order to ensure the client could remain at home.

8. This is not to say that rules don't matter, but technical rules can be far too limiting. Nevertheless, there are general principles that refer to rights and distributive justice (or what people owe one another). I will say more about this in chapters 3 and 4.

9. Ironically, as I am arguing, by discouraging aides from forming bonds with clients, agencies are creating the very burnout conditions that they want to avoid, since it results in high employee turnover. Study after study shows that aides find the personal relationships formed to be the most fulfilling aspect of the home care aide job.

10. I say "a" philosophy because this is an issue that needs further consideration beyond the pages of this book; the philosophy I am offering here is just one of many possibilities. If I argued for "the" philosophy of home care, my position would take on the trappings of a unitary, all-inclusive worldview. But this is not what I intend. Rather, I would imagine that philosophies of home care will differ from culture to culture, depending on different ways of life and social and economic resources. The model I am suggesting is specifically aimed at the United States and Canada. While Canada has a system of universal health care, the same kinds of cultural assumptions and ideologies are at work in the home care setting.

### 3. Women's Care Work as a Subsidy to the State

1. As Mary Romero puts it, "The dependency of a Rockefeller toddler or sick aging member of the Rockefeller clan is not the same as the dependency of a toddler or chronically ill parent of a secretary, waitress, sales clerk, nurse, or teacher" (2000, 188).

2. Other feminist approaches to moral theory include Habermasian discourse ethics, liberal, and deontological ethics. In this chapter I will focus on an ethic of care; chapter 5 will consider how discourse ethics can serve to democratize home care.

3. The notion of a "care" perspective derives from Carol Gilligan (1982). Gilligan posits two ways of moral reasoning that can be roughly attributed to men and women. She points out that men tend to reason from a "justice" perspective, where they focus on rights, justice, and abstract moral principles, and that women tend to reason from a "care" perspective, where their concern is with maintaining relationships, nurturing and caring for others, and being responsive to the details of each situation.

4. Gilligan identified this "ethic of care" in response to the work of Lawrence Kohlberg, a moral development theorist who argued that women are largely incapable of reaching the highest stages of moral development. Kohlberg conducted studies that showed boys' ability to reach the highest stages of moral development (that is, the capacity to reason impartially, based on abstract rules/principles such as justice) and that showed girls' widespread incapacity to think independently outside of particular relationships. Gilligan indicates that the girls in Kohlberg's study were

merely using a "different voice" to identify the moral features of a situation: the "care" voice.

5. Note that Gilligan does not posit an essentialist notion of women as "care" ethicists and men as "justice" ethicists. On the contrary, she suggests that gender role socialization may be the cause of these gendered ways of moral reasoning; furthermore, she suggests that some men may reason from an ethic of care while some women may reason from a justice perspective.

6. For feminist philosophers' accounts of the ethic of care, see Held (1987), Grimshaw (1986), Kittay and Meyers (1987), Walker (1998), Tronto (1993), and Noddings (1984).

7. This critique of governments covers a number of countries, including (but not limited to) England, Canada, and the United States.

8. According to Marilyn Frye (1984), what makes a practice oppressive is its connection to other practices, policies, and beliefs that limit the freedoms of individuals (or groups of individuals). So, for example, home care—in its current state— is oppressive for women because its practice is rooted within a system of interlocking barriers that limit women's options and freedoms.

9. My home care supervisor was of little help under these circumstances: She would tell me to "just go home" since my shift was over. In talking to other home care aides, I discovered (unsurprisingly) that I was not alone in putting in extra, unpaid hours; home health care's fiscal viability is thus largely based on the unpaid, unrecognized labor of female family members *and* home care aides.

10. I say "less" exploitative and alienating because I believe home health care will always exploit and alienate female caregivers to some degree. At best, we can render it as minimally exploitative and alienating as possible.

11. Kittay (1999) refers to a "pubic ethic of care."

12. For more on relational autonomy, see chapter 4.

13. I do not distinguish here between marketized and socialized systems of health care, since both types of systems emphasize values of autonomy, independence, and impartiality, and both fail to satisfactorily address the subordination of women and minorities.

14. For a good discussion of how autonomy came to be the guiding principle of health care ethics, see Wolpe (1998).

15. Given my critique of home health care, that individuals prefer home care to institutional care is historically contingent on our hyper-valuing of autonomy and independence. Long-term care facilities could be desirable places to go if we put more emphasis on chronic and long-term care and if we did not so strongly privilege autonomy and independence.

16. Susan Moller Okin (1989) has criticized Rawls for limiting his focus to the sphere of public, political interactions. She has written extensively on the need for justice in the family, since the family is one of the primary social institutions. Okin argues that, to ensure gender equality among those sharing a household, any comprehensive theory of justice must ensure that justice also pertains within the family.

17. See Kittay (1999) for a discussion of "nested dependencies."

18. Economists understand efficiency in terms of "pareto efficiency." On this notion, as long as everyone benefits, and no one is hurt, an unequal distribution is efficient.

19. Work that involves heavy lifting, distasteful jobs (like collecting garbage, tarring roofs, etc.), and/or dangerous work sites (working on high-rise buildings as a window washer, construction work, or mining) is usually well paid because of the dangers and distastefulness inherent to the job. This is not so in the case of home care aides, despite the heavy lifting of clients that is involved, the distasteful job of cleaning up urine, feces, vomit, etc., and the sometimes dangerous neighborhoods and homes that aides are expected to enter to complete their work.

20. Of course, home care *is* extremely valuable work. As I have been arguing, and as Kittay (1997, 1999) and Fineman (2000) argue, caretaking work is foundational to a well-functioning, rationally organized, caring society. But I think it is a separate question as to whether the actual value of one's work is recognized as *being* valuable.

21. The move in some states toward paid family caretaking may bring even closer together the issues for family caretakers and those for formal, paid caretakers. Whether or not paid family caretaking is an effective, efficient way for the state to provide home care services is a point of serious contention among home care theorists.

22. And even animal workers receive more pay than home care workers—a fact which should make one question what this tells us about how we value persons receiving home care.

23. See, for example, Donovan (1989), Feldman (1997), and Chichin (1992).

24. For a good critique of the view of physicians as hired hands or plumbers, see Veatch (1972).

25. Catriona Mackenzie (2000) and Diana Meyers (2000) have used this terminology in their work on moral imagination.

26. Vincent Schodolski, "Union Signals a Health Trend," *Chicago Tribune*, February 26, 1999. While Medicare and Medicaid caps on reimbursement for home care services keep home care wages low, agencies could raise wages and offer benefits to workers and still make a profit. Just how much room there is for wage increases is another contentious issue.

27. Stone and Yamada (1998, 46).

## 4. Caring about the Cared-For

1. In *Love's Labor,* Kittay makes her arguments with an eye to the most dependent citizens, those who cannot reciprocate care at all. As she claims, "I begin with the case of a dependent who is unable to reciprocate not because I assume it to be a most typical case, but because it is the case most in need of consideration if one is asking about the social responsibility to the caregiver. That social responsibility diminishes as the dependent is more and more capable of reciprocating and as the dependent is less than totally helpless. The less helpless and more capable the dependent, the closer the relationship begins to approximate relations between equals" (1999, xiii). Similarly, in this chapter I begin with the frail, dependent, elderly female because she is the most typical case in home care and also because it leads us to the most pressing questions about organizing home health care.

2. See Golden and Sonneborn (1998), Brickner (1997), and Post (1995). For work that focuses on ageist attitudes against elderly women, see Arber and Ginn (1991), Pearsall (1997), Greer (1993), and Walker (1999).

3. Consider one of my home care clients, who was 80, yet distanced herself from her own age by referring to her "elderly brother," who was 84; furthermore, the lengths to which aging citizens will go to stave off aging (through face lifts, vitamins, and enhancement technologies) indicates a rejection of aging.

4. For an interesting discussion of aging women and physical appearance, see Meyers (1999).

5. "Caring for Ailing Aged Linked to Strain, Death," *Chicago Tribune,* December 15, 1999.

6. This is not to suggest that I did not witness a great deal of altruism in my home care work. Friends and neighbors brought meals, news, and conversational tidbits to my home-bound clients. I did note, however, that such altruism became strained over time, as visitors felt the pressure of their own personal and work commitments.

7. For more on this issue of women's self-regarding choices, see Parks (2000).

8. This is why I am arguing for a melding of care and justice. Just as we can have too much care in home care, we can focus too much on individual rights and independence. My home care client's refusal to bathe seriously affected her overall care, and her bodily odor sickened the aides, thus minimizing their social contact with her.

9. Not all home care theorists agree on the importance of accommodation over autonomy. For a criticism of "accommodating" elderly home care recipients, see Fiore (1999).

10. My concern here is not rationing care because of its cost. But I do think that applying high-tech care to clients with very poor long-term prognoses is unwise and may even be cruel, since such measures may serve to prolong a life of physical and emotional pain and suffering.

11. As William Ruddick (1995) has noted, such high-tech interventions may also impact the families of home care clients, turning their homes into institution-like places and often alienating them from it.

12. Of course, such tethering to our identities can sometimes prove problematic when families persist in associating us with selves that we can no longer identify with. Sometimes families saddle us with the responsibility to be who we once were but who we can no longer be because of illness or disability.

### 5. The Personal Is Political

1. Eva Kittay (1999) points out that some cared-for cannot reciprocate in any way, not even by recognizing the care given by others. In such cases, reciprocity is strained. In other cases (like one's relationship with a garage mechanic), reciprocity is formal and accountable: Each party expects something from the other. Experiences in the home care setting can vary on a continuum from one extreme to another.

2. The term *emboldened autonomy* is coined by Collopy, Dubler, and Zuckerman (1990) in their work on home care. By virtue of being in the familiarity and comfort of their homes, clients may become "emboldened" in their attempts at autonomy. Such emboldened autonomy is expressed, for example, in the refusal to take medications or accept care by caretakers.

3. Note that requests for certain kinds of workers may not be fulfilled simply because a person of the desired background may not be available. A racist client

may not want a black woman in her home, but she may have to be willing to accept the services of a black worker or forfeit home care altogether. Thus, practical considerations could limit clients' demands for home care aides of a particular race or ethnic background.

4. "Home Health Care in Crisis: Criminal Caregivers," *Record,* October 3, 1999.

5. "The Unlicensed Underground," *Record,* October 10, 1999.

6. As Alasdair MacIntyre (2000) has indicated, we ought to develop a standard of care before we look to economic questions. Rather than allowing our economic situation to determine what care we can afford to supply, he argues that as a community we ought to develop a standard and *then* consider how we will meet it.

7. By "ontological space," I mean a place that is foundational to the very constitution of an individual's self.

8. I say "decent" because I assert that, even if a client might receive *better* care in an institution, this should not settle the case of whether she is transferred to one. What really matters is whether she can still get decent care at home; if so, then there must be other reasons for moving her.

9. This does not mean that we should use an individual's lack of relationships to justify taking her out of her home. Just because a person is living alone, isolated, and largely out of contact doesn't mean that an agency has reason to institutionalize that person. On the contrary, if the individual identifies herself as a "loner" who has never enjoyed the company of others, and if she prefers a life of solitude, then we also have good relational reasons for respecting that preference.

10. See Holstein and Mitzen (2001). Thanks to David Ingram for helping me to think through this section of the book.

11. Ingram uses the term *affirmative remedies* to designate "those remedies that work within the systemic and identity-based injustices of our current society" (2000, 44).

12. Some bioethicists refer explicitly to the work of Habermas; many others implicitly assume the value of a communicative ethic in health care. In an explicit appeal to Habermas, bioethicist Harry Moody (1992) claims, "I am trying to argue, in the tradition of Dewey or Habermas, that unless we understand the pragmatic origins and the consequences of our ideas, we will fail to make our ideas clear to those who must act in the world. The result of failure is that theory and practice, ethics and politics, remain estranged and communication remains blocked."

13. For example, see Benhabib (1996b) and Fleming (1997).

## 6. Looking Ahead

1. As one study notes, low back injuries are predominant among home care workers and even surpass the rate of worker injury in hospital settings. For incidents where patients were being handled, in 88 percent of cases the home care aide was working alone, compared with 39 percent in the institution. As Myers, Jensen et al. claim, "In the home, the following factors could contribute to the risk of back injury: the lower height of beds, lack of height adjustability, access to beds, a greater likelihood of working without the possibility of getting help with heavy tasks, and unavailability of patient handling equipment such as patient lifts and transfer devices" (1993, 150).

2. For an extended discussion on the importance of discourse to home care provision, see chapter 5.

3. The quotes that follow are taken from an Access Living focus group on personal assistants that was held on March 5, 2001. The interview was done through the Center for Urban Research and Learning (CURL) at Loyola University of Chicago.

4. For example, the California In-Home Supportive Services program is one of the most successful independent provider programs in the United States. Studies from the 1980s indicate that service costs for independent providers in the California program were 55 percent lower than those of home care agencies. But these savings are created by offering lower wages and benefits for workers. See Feldman (1997) and Feldman, Sapienza, and Kane (1990).

5. By contrast, some supporters see independent provider programs in California and Wisconsin as success stories.

6. These 75,000 are in addition to the more than 80,000 home care workers who already belonged to SEIU nationwide. The addition of the California home care workers means that SEIU now has 1.3 million home care workers as members. See Vincent Schodolski, "Union Signals a Health Trend," *Chicago Tribune,* February 26, 1999.

7. "Agency Lets Aides Hold Their Destiny," *Record,* October 17, 1999.

8. For an excellent account of worker-managed firms, see Schweickart (1993, 99ff.).

9. I am not trying to deny a place for privacy, or personal concerns over which politics should not have control. I still think that women's abortion choices, for example, are personal, private ones with which the state should not interfere. But notice that they are nevertheless public choices insofar as women require the public provision of abortion clinics in order to make the personal choice.

10. This is similar to Diana Meyers's conception of "autonomy competency" in *Self, Society, and Personal Choice* (1989). Meyers sees autonomy as having both social and natural components, and she argues that individuals should be encouraged to develop as much as possible their capacity for autonomy.

11. In some cases, the care recipient may be so profoundly dependent that she cannot formulate her own conception of the good. In such cases, I would argue, those who identify with and through their charges—mothers, caretakers—are best suited to formulating that conception for the dependent person.

12. MacIntyre approvingly refers to the Supreme Court *Olmstead* decision. In this case, the Court denied the state of Georgia's discriminatory practice of making the availability of mental health services contingent on an individual's residing in an institution. While MacIntyre agrees with the Court's decision, he argues that we cannot continue to make such decisions absent a clear standard of care. As he says, "Once we have . . . a standard of care governing how we act toward the mentally retarded and mentally ill, then it is indeed important that that standard is applied in a nondiscriminatory way. But no prohibition of discriminatory conduct will itself yield a standard of care" (2000, 82).

13. See Daniels (1985, 1993, 2000). While the capabilities approach and Daniels's notion of a "normal opportunity range" may be problematic because of their reliance on biological characteristics, I do think they are appropriate to this context. We need institutions that will transform primary goods into capabilities for

individuals. I will leave aside the issue of whether capabilities are naturally given, a controversial issue that has divided disability theorists into the social versus the medical model of disability. For my purposes, Sen's capabilities model gets at the importance of doing more than throwing money at deep problems with our social and political arrangement.

14. Thanks to Alexandre de Miranda for making this observation.

15. See Callahan (1999); Angell (1997); Brickner (1997).

# WORKS CITED

Abel, Emily K. 1997. "Adult Daughters and Care for the Elderly." In *The Other Within Us: Feminist Explorations of Women and Aging,* ed. Marilyn Pearsall, 135–50. Boulder, Colo.: Westview Press.

Angell, Marcia. 1997. "Fixing Medicare." *New England Journal of Medicine* 337 (3): 192–94.

Arber, Sara, and Jay Ginn. 1991. *Gender and Later Life.* London: Sage.

Arno, Peter S., Carol Levine, and Margaret M. Memmott. 1999. "The Economic Value of Informal Caregiving." *Health Affairs* 18 (2): 182–88.

Aronson, Jane. 1992. "Women's Sense of Responsibility for the Care of Old People: 'But Who Else Is Going to Do It?'" *Gender and Society* 6 (1): 8–29.

Asch, Adrienne. 1993. "Free to Be a Bigot." In *Ethical Conflicts in the Management of Home Care,* ed. Rosalie Kane and Arthur Caplan, 223–31. New York: Springer.

Baier, Annette. 1985. *Postures of the Mind: Essays on Mind and Morals.* Minneapolis: University of Minnesota Press.

Barclay, Linda. 2000. "Autonomy and the Social Self." In *Relational Autonomy: Feminist Perspectives on Autonomy, Agency, and the Social Self,* ed. Catriona Mackenzie and Natalie Stoljar, 52–71. New York: Oxford University Press.

Bartky, Sandra Lee. 1999. "Unplanned Obsolescence: Some Reflections on Aging." In *Mother Time: Women, Aging, and Ethics,* ed. Margaret Walker, 61–74. New York: Rowman and Littlefield.

Bayles, Michael. 1988. "The Professions." In *Ethical Issues in Professional Life,* ed. Joan Callahan, 27–31. New York: Oxford University Press.

Beauchamp, Tom, and James Childress. 2001. *Principles of Biomedical Ethics.* 5th ed. New York: Oxford University Press.

Beauvoir, Simone de. 1980. *The Second Sex,* translated by H. M. Parshley. 1952; rpt., New York: Knopf.

Bell, Nora Kizer. 1992. "If Age Becomes a Standard for Rationing Health Care . . ." In *Feminist Perspectives in Medical Ethics,* ed. Helen Bequaert Holmes and Laura M. Purdy, 83–90. Bloomington: Indiana University Press.

Benhabib, Seyla. 1987. "The Generalized and the Concrete Other: The Kohlberg-Gilligan Controversy and Moral Theory." In *Women and Moral Theory,* ed. Eva Kittay and Diana Meyers, 154–77. Totowa, N.J.: Rowman and Littlefield.

———. 1996a. "Autonomy, Modernity and Community: Communitarianism and Critical Social Theory in Dialogue." In *Social Justice in a Diverse Society,* ed. Rita Manning and Ruth Trujillo, 75–83. Mountain View, Calif.: Mayfield.

———, ed. 1996b. *Democracy and Difference: Contesting the Boundaries of the Political.* Princeton, N.J.: Princeton University Press.

Blackwell, James. 1985. *The Black Community: Diversity and Unity.* New York: Dodd, Mead.

Blaser, Jean. 1998. "The Case Against Paid Family Caregivers: Ethical and Practical Issues." *Generations* 22 (3): 65–69.

Brickner, Philip W. 1997. "Long-Term Home Health Care for the Frail Aged." In *Geriatric Home Health Care,* ed. Philip W. Brickner, F. Russell Kellogg, Anthony J. Lechich, Roberta Lipsman, and Linda K. Scharer, 41–57. New York: Springer.

Brison, Susan. 1997. "Outliving Oneself: Trauma, Memory, and Personal Identity." In *Feminists Rethink the Self,* ed. Diana Meyers, 12–39. Boulder, Colo.: Westview Press.

Butler, Judith. 1990. *Gender Trouble: Feminism and the Subversion of Identity.* New York: Routledge.

Callahan, Daniel. 1999. "Age, Sex, and Resource Allocation." In *Mother Time: Women, Aging, and Ethics,* ed. Margaret Walker, 189–99. New York: Rowman and Littlefield.

Chichin, Eileen R. 1992. "Home Care Is Where the Heart Is: The Role of Interpersonal Relationships in Paraprofessional Home Care." *Home Health Care Services Quarterly* 13 (1–2): 161–77.

Christiansen, Kathryn. 1995. "A Paradigm Shift for the Home Care Provider." In *Home Care and Managed Care: Strategies for the Future,* ed. Eric Linne, 13–19. Chicago: American Hospital.

Collopy, Bart. 1990. "An Introduction to Home Care: What Are the Issues?" In *Home Health Care Options,* ed. Connie Zuckerman, Nancy Dubler, and Bart Collopy, 3–23. New York: Plenum Press.

Collopy, Bart, Nancy Dubler, and Connie Zuckerman. 1990. "The Ethics of Home Care: Autonomy and Accommodation." *Hastings Center Report,* March.

Dalley, Gillian. 1984. "Ideologies of Care: A Feminist Contribution to the Debate." *Critical Social Policy* 8: 72–81.

Daniels, Norman. 1985. *Just Health Care.* New York: Cambridge University Press.

———. 1993. "Rationing Fairly: Programmatic Considerations." *Bioethics* 7 (2–3): 224–33.

———. 2000. "Mental Disabilities, Equal Opportunity and the ADA." In *Americans with Disabilities: Exploring Implications of the Law for Individuals and Institutions,* ed. Leslie Pickering Francis and Anita Silvers, 255–66. New York: Routledge.

Donovan, Rebecca. 1989. "Work Stress and Job Satisfaction: A Study of Home Care Workers in New York City." *Home Health Services Quarterly* 10: 97–114.

Dubler, Nancy Neveloff. 1990. "Accommodating the Home Care Client: A Look at Rights and Interests." In *Home Health Care Options,* ed. Connie Zuckerman, Nancy Dubler, and Bart Collopy, 141–65. New York: Insight Books.

Ehrenreich, Barbara, and Deirdre English. 1989. *For Her Own Good: 150 Years of the Experts' Advice to Women.* New York: Doubleday.

Feder, Judith, Harriet Komisar, and Marlene Niefeld. 2000. "Long-Term Care in the United States: An Overview." *Health Affairs* 19 (3): 40–56.

Feldman, Penny Hollander. 1997. "Labor Market Issues in Home Care." In *Home-Based Care for a New Century,* ed. Daniel Fox and Carol Raphael, 155–83. Malden, Mass.: Blackwell.

Feldman, Penny Hollander, Alice M. Sapienza, and Nancy M. Kane. 1990. *Who Cares for Them: Workers in the Home Care Industry.* New York: Greenwood Press.

Finch, Janet. 1984. "Community Care: Developing Non-Sexist Alternatives." *Critical Social Policy* 9: 16–18.

Finch, Janet, and Dulcie Groves. 1983. *A Labor of Love: Women, Work, and Caring.* London: Routledge and Kegan Paul.

Fineman, Martha. 2000. "Cracking the Foundational Myths: Independence, Autonomy, and Self-Sufficiency." *American Journal of Gender, Social Policy, and the Law* 8 (13): 12–29.

Fiore, Robin. 1999. "Caring for Ourselves: Peer Care in Autonomous Aging." In *Mother Time: Women, Aging, and Ethics,* ed. Margaret Walker, 245–60. New York: Rowman and Littlefield.

Fisk, Milton. 2000. *Toward a Healthy Society: The Morality and Politics of American Health Care Reform.* Lawrence: University Press of Kansas.

Fleming, Marie. 1997. *Emancipation and Illusion: Rationality and Gender in Habermas's Theory of Modernity.* University Park: Pennsylvania State University Press.

Folbre, Nancy, and Ann Ferguson. 2000. "Women, Care, and the Public Good: A Dialogue." In *Not for Sale: In Defence of Public Goods,* ed. Anatole Anton, Milton Fisk, and Nancy Holmstrom, 95–107. Boulder, Colo.: Westview Press.

Frank, Arthur. 1991. *At the Will of the Body: Reflections on Illness.* Boston: Houghton Mifflin.

Franklin, John Hope, and Eleanor Holmes Norton. 1987. *Black Initiative and Governmental Responsibility: A Policy Framework for Racial Justice.* Washington, D.C.: Joint Center for Political Studies.

Friedman, Marilyn. 1993. *What Are Friends For?* Ithaca, N.Y.: Cornell University Press.

Frye, Marilyn. 1984. *The Politics of Reality.* Trumansburg, N.Y.: Crossing Press.

Gilligan, Carol. 1982. *In a Different Voice: Psychological Theory and Women's Development.* Cambridge, Mass.: Harvard University Press.

———. 1987. "Moral Orientation and Moral Development." In *Women and Moral Theory,* ed. Eva Kittay and Diana Meyers, 19–33. Totowa: Rowman and Littlefield.

Golden, Robyn L., and Sallie Sonneborn. 1998. "Ethics in Clinical Practice with Older Adults: Recognizing Biases and Respecting Boundaries." *Generations* 22 (3): 82–86

Graham, Hilary. 1983. "Caring: A Labour of Love." In *A Labour of Love: Women, Work, and Caring,* ed. Janet Finch and Dulcie Groves, 13–30. London: Routledge and Kegan Paul.

Greer, Germaine. 1993. *The Change: Women, Aging, and the Menopause.* New York: Fawcett Books.

Grimshaw, Jean. 1986. *Philosophy and Feminist Thinking.* Minneapolis: University of Minnesota Press.

Habermas, Jürgen. 1989–90. "Justice and Solidarity: On the Discussion Concerning 'Stage 6.'" *Philosophical Forum* 21: 32–52.

———. 1990. "Discourse Ethics: Notes on a Program of Philosophical Justification." In *The Communicative Ethics Controversy,* ed. Seyla Benhabib and Fred Dallmayr. Cambridge: MIT Press.

Held, Virginia. 1987. "Non-contractual Society: A Feminist View." *Canadian Journal of Philosophy* 13: 111–37.

Hinton-Walker, P. 1993. "Care of the Chronically Ill: Paradigm Shifts and Directions for the Future." *Holistic Nursing Practice* 8 (1): 56–66.

Hobbes, Thomas. 1968. *Leviathan.* Ed. C. B. Macpherson. 1651; rpt., New York: Penguin Books.

Holstein, Martha. 1999. "Home Care, Women, and Aging: A Case Study of Injustice." In *Mother Time: Women, Aging, and Ethics,* ed. Margaret Walker, 227–44. New York: Rowman and Littlefield.

Holstein, Martha, and Phyllis Mitzen, eds. 2001. *Ethics in Community-Based Elder Care.* New York: Springer.

Houston, Barbara. 1987. "Rescuing Womanly Virtues: Some Dangers of Moral Reclamation." *Canadian Journal of Philosophy* 13: 237–62.

Hudson, Robert B. 1990. "Home Care Policy: Loved by All, Feared by Many." In *Home Health Care Options,* ed. Connie Zuckerman, Nancy Dubler, and Bart Collopy, 271–301. New York: Insight Books.

Ingram, David. 1990. *Critical Theory and Philosophy.* New York: Paragon House.

———. 2000. *Group Rights: Reconciling Equality and Difference.* Lawrence: University Press of Kansas.

Jennings, Bruce, Daniel Callahan, and Arthur Caplan. 1988. "Ethical Challenges of Chronic Illness." *Hastings Center Report,* February/March, 1–16.

Kane, Rosalie, and Arthur Caplan, eds. 1993. *Ethical Conflicts in the Management of Home Care.* New York: Springer.

Kane, Rosalie, and Carrie Levin. 1998. "Who's Safe? Who's Sorry? The Duty to Protect the Safety of Clients in Home- and Community-Based Care." *Generations* 22 (3): 76–81.

Kant, Immanuel. 1990. *Foundations for the Metaphysics of Morals.* 2d ed. Translated from the 1785 original by Lewis White Beck. New York: Macmillan, Library of the Liberal Arts.

Karner, Tracy X. 1998. "Professional Caring: Homecare Workers as Fictive Kin." *Journal of Aging Studies* 12: 69–83.

Kaye, Lenard W. 1992. *Home Health Care.* Newbury Park, Calif.: Sage.

Kayser-Jones, Jeanie. 1995. "High-Tech Home Care for Elderly Persons: Issues and Recommendations." In *Bringing the Hospital Home,* ed. John Arras, 129–45. Baltimore: Johns Hopkins University Press.

Kittay, Eva. 1997. "Human Dependency and Rawlsian Equality." In *Feminists Rethink the Self,* ed. Diana Meyers, 219–66. Boulder, Colo.: Westview Press.

———. 1999. *Love's Labor: Essays on Women, Equality, and Dependency.* New York: Routledge.

———. 2000. "At Home with My Daughter." In *Americans with Disabilities: Exploring Implications of the Law for Individuals and Institutions,* ed. Leslie Pickering Francis and Anita Silvers, 64–80. New York: Routledge.

Kittay, Eva, and Diana Meyers, eds. 1987. *Women and Moral Theory.* Totowa, N.J.: Rowman and Littlefield.

Kuhse, Helga. 1997. *Caring: Nurses, Women, and Ethics,* Malden, Mass.: Blackwell.

Kuttner, Robert. 1997. *Everything for Sale.* New York: Alfred A. Knopf.

Layton, Mary Jo, and Thomas Zambito. 1999. "Home Health Care in Crisis: Criminal Caregivers," <http://199.173.2.7/news/smainbar199910031.htm>, and "The Unlicensed Underground," <http://199.173.2.7/news/day2main199910101.htm>.

Linne, Eric. 1995. "Home Care and Managed Care: The Future Approaches." In *Home Care and Managed Care: Strategies for the Future,* ed. Eric Linne, 1–12. Chicago: American Hospital.

MacIntyre, Alasdair. 2000. "The Need for a Standard of Care." In *Americans with Disabilities: Exploring Implications of the Law for Individuals and Institutions,* ed. Leslie Pickering Francis and Anita Silvers, 81–86. New York: Routledge.

Mackenzie, Catriona. 2000. "Imagining Oneself Otherwise." In *Relational Autonomy: Feminist Perspectives on Autonomy, Agency, and the Social Self,* ed. Catriona Mackenzie and Natalie Stoljar, 124–50. New York: Oxford University Press.

MacKinnon, Catharine. 1989. *Toward a Feminist Theory of the State.* Cambridge, Mass.: Harvard University Press.

Mahowald, Mary, Anita Silvers, and David Wasserman. 1998. "A Feminist Standpoint." In *Disability, Difference, Discrimination: Perspectives on Justice in Bioethics and Public Policy.* New York: Rowman and Littlefield.

McCluskey, Martha T. 2000. "Subsidized Lives and the Ideology of Efficiency." *American University Journal of Gender, Social Policy, and the Law* 8: 115–54.

Meyers, Diana. 1989. *Self, Society, and Personal Choice.* New York: Columbia University Press.

———. 1999. "Miroir, Memoire, Mirage: Appearance, Aging, and Women." In *Mother Time: Women, Aging, and Ethics,* ed. Margaret Urban Walker, 23–41. New York: Rowman and Littlefield.

———. 2000. "Intersectional Identity and the Authentic Self? Opposites Attract!" In *Relational Autonomy: Feminist Perspectives on Autonomy, Agency, and the Social Self,* ed. Catriona Mackenzie and Natalie Stoljar, 151–80. New York: Oxford University Press.

Mill, John Stuart. 1957. *Utilitarianism.* 1861; rpt., Indianapolis: Bobbs-Merrill.

Minow, Martha. 1990. *Making All the Difference: Inclusion, Exclusion, and American Law.* Ithaca: Cornell University Press.

Moody, Harry. 1992. *Ethics in an Aging Society.* Baltimore: Johns Hopkins University Press.

Moros, D., R. Rhodes, B. Baumrin, and J. Strain. 1991. "Chronic Illness and the Physician-Patient Relationship: A Response to the Hastings Center's 'Ethical Challenges of Chronic Illness.'" *Journal of Medicine and Philosophy* 16: 161–81.

Myers, Ann, Roger C. Jensen, David Nestor, and Jacqueline Rattiner. 1993. "Low Back Injuries among Home Health Aides Compared with Hospital Nursing Aides." *Home Health Care Services Quarterly* 14: 149–55.

Nelson, James Lindemann. 2002. "Just Expectations: Family Caregivers, Practical Identities, and Social Justice in the Provision of Health Care." In *Medicine and Social Justice,* ed. Rhodes, Battin, and Silvers. Cambridge: Oxford University Press. In press.

Nelson, James Lindemann, and Hilde Lindemann Nelson. 1995. *The Patient in the Family: An Ethics of Medicine and Families.* New York: Routledge.

Noddings, Nel. 1984. *Caring: A Feminine Approach to Ethics and Moral Education.* Berkeley: University of California Press.

———. 1995. "Moral Obligations or Moral Support for High-Tech Home Care?" In *Bringing the Hospital Home,* ed. John Arras, 149–65. Baltimore: Johns Hopkins University Press.

———. 1996. "The Cared-For." In *Caregiving: Readings in Knowledge, Practice, Ethics, and Politics,* ed. Suzanne Gordon, Patricia Benner, and Nel Noddings, 21–39. Philadelphia: University of Pennsylvania Press.

Okin, Susan Moller. 1989. *Justice, Gender and the Family.* New York: Basic Books.

Ontario Ministry of Health. 1992. *Managing Health Care Resources.* Toronto: Publications Ontario.

Ozar, David, and David Sokol. 1994. *Dental Ethics at Chairside.* St. Louis: Mosby.

Parks, Jennifer. 2000. "Why Gender Matters to the Euthanasia Debate: On Decisional Capacity and the Rejection of Women's Death Requests." *Hastings Center Report* 30 (1): 32–39.

Pearsall, Marilyn, ed. 1997. *The Other Within Us: Feminist Explorations of Women and Aging.* Boulder, Colo.: Westview Press.

Perry, Twila. 2000. "Caretakers, Entitlement, and Diversity." *American University Journal of Gender, Social Policy, and the Law* 8: 153–64.

Post, Stephen. 1995. *The Moral Challenge of Alzheimer Disease.* Baltimore: Johns Hopkins University Press.

Pousada, Lidia. 1995. "High-Tech Home Care for Elderly Persons: What, Why, and How Much?" In *Bringing the Hospital Home,* ed. John Arras, 107–28. Baltimore: Johns Hopkins University Press.

Prado, Carlos. 2000. *Starting with Foucault.* 2d ed. Boulder, Colo.: Westview Press.

Rawls, John. 1971. *A Theory of Justice.* Cambridge, Mass.: Harvard University Press.

———. 1980. "Kantian Constructivism in Moral Theory: The Dewey Lectures 1980." *Journal of Philosophy* 77 (9): 515–72.

Reinharz, Shulamit. 1997. "Friends or Foes: Gerontological and Feminist Theory." In *The Other Within Us: Feminist Explorations of Women and Aging,* ed. Marilyn Pearsall. Boulder, Colo.: Westview Press.

Roberts, Dorothy. 1997. *Killing the Black Body: Race, Reproduction, and the Meaning of Liberty.* New York: Pantheon Books.

Romero, Mary. 2000. "Bursting the Foundational Myths of Reproductive Labor Under Capitalism: A Call for Brave New Families or Brave New Villages?" *American University Journal of Gender, Social Policy, and the Law* 8: 181–94.

Roth, P., and J. Harrison. 1991. "Orchestrating Social Change: An Imperative in the Care of the Chronically Ill." *Journal of Medicine and Philosophy* 16: 343–59.

Ruddick, Sara. 1989. *Maternal Thinking.* New York: Ballantine Books.

Ruddick, William. 1995. "Transforming Homes and Hospitals." In *Bringing the Hospital Home,* ed. John Arras, 166–79. Baltimore: Johns Hopkins University Press.

Scharer, Linda K. 1997. "Informal Supports." In *Geriatric Home Health Care,* ed. Philip W. Brickner, F. Russell Kellogg, Anthony J. Lechich, Roberta Lipsman, and Linda K. Scharer, 41–57. New York: Springer.

Schultz, Vicki. 2000. "Life's Work." *Columbia Law Review* 100: 1881–1963.

Schweickart, David. 1993. *Against Capitalism.* Cambridge: Cambridge University Press.

Sen, Amartya. 1990. "Justice: Means versus Freedoms." *Philosophy and Public Affairs* 19 (2): 111–21.

Sherwin, Susan. 1992. *No Longer Patient: Feminist Ethics and Health Care.* Philadelphia: Temple University Press.

Silvers, Anita, David Wasserman, and Mary Mahowald. 1998. "Formal Justice." In *Disability, Difference, Discrimination: Perspectives on Justice in Bioethics and Public Policy.* New York: Rowman and Littlefield.

Simon-Rusinowitz, Lori, Kevin J. Mahoney, and A. E. Benjamin. 1998. "Payments to Families Who Provide Care: An Option That Should Be Available." *Generations* 22 (3): 69–75.

Stone, Robyn I., and Yoshiko Yamada. 1998. "Ethics and the Frontline Long-Term-Care Worker: A Challenge for the Twenty-first Century." *Generations* 22 (3): 45–51.

Strickling, Bonelle Lewis. 1988. "Self-Abnegation." In *Feminist Perspectives: Philosophical Essays on Method and Morals,* ed. Lorraine Code, Sheila Mullett, and Christine Overall, 190–201. Toronto: University of Toronto Press.

Tronto, Joan. 1993. *Moral Boundaries: A Political Argument for an Ethic of Care.* New York: Routledge.

———. 1998. "An Ethic of Care." *Generations* 22 (3): 15–20.

Veatch, Robert. 1972. "Models for Ethical Practice in a Revolutionary Age." *Hastings Center Report* 2 (3): 5–7.

Walker, Alan. 1983. "Care for Elderly People: A Conflict between Women and the State." In *A Labour of Love: Women, Work, and Caring,* ed. Janet Finch and Dulcie Groves, 106–28. London: Routledge and Kegan Paul.

Walker, Margaret Urban. 1998. *Moral Understandings: A Study in Feminist Ethics.* New York: Routledge.

———, ed. 1999. *Mother Time: Women, Aging, and Ethics.* New York: Rowman and Littlefield.

Waymack, Mark. 2001. "The Ethical Importance of Home Care." In *Ethics and Community-Based Elder Care,* ed. Martha Holstein and Phyllis Mitzen, 51–59. New York: Springer.

Wendell, Susan. 1992. "Toward a Feminist Theory of Disability." In *Feminist Perspectives in Medical Ethics,* ed. Helen Bequaert Holmes and Laura M. Purdy, 63–81. Bloomington: Indiana University Press.

Williams, Oliver J. 1993. "When Is Being Equal Unfair?" In *Ethical Conflicts in the Management of Home Care,* ed. Rosalie Kane and Arthur Caplan, 206–15. New York: Springer.

Wolf, Susan. 1996. *Feminism and Bioethics: Beyond Reproduction.* New York: Oxford University Press.

Wolpe, Paul Root. 1998. "The Triumph of Autonomy in American Bioethics: A Sociological View." In *Bioethics and Society: Constructing the Ethical Enterprise,* ed. Raymond DeVries and Janardan Subedi, 38–59. Upper Saddle River, N.J.: Prentice Hall.

Zuckerman, Connie, Nancy Dubler, and Bart Collopy, eds. 1990. *Home Health Care Options.* New York: Plenum Press.

# INDEX

Abel, Emily, 54
abuse, 1, 2; clients, 47–48, 100–104; home
  care system, 101
Asch, Adrienne, 98
autonomy, 5, 23–25, 42, 60–61, 112, 132,
  143n7; emboldened, 97, 149n2; independence, 60–61; relational, 5, 7, 9–10,
  17, 85–88, 90, 92, 144nn10,11; self-control, 22

Baier, Annette, 86
Barclay, Linda, 86
Bartky, Sandra, 75
Bayles, Michael, 37
Beauchamp, James, and James Childress,
  100. See also justice, non-maleficence
Beauvoir, Simone de, 145n12
Bell, Nora Kizer, 4
Benhabib, Seyla, 40
Blackwell, James, 26
Blaser, Jean, 109–111
Brickner, Philip, 141
Brison, Susan, 87

Callahan, Daniel, 23
capabilities, 16, 133–135. See also Sen,
  Amartya
Caplan, Arthur, 23
care: acute, 22–25, 41–42, 49, 144n9; activities and instrumental activities of daily
  living (ADLs and IADLs), 2, 5, 8, 17, 19,
  52, 145n17; chronic, 22–25; community-
  based, 10–11, 20, 143n4; criminal,
  101–103; decubitus, 81–82; family,
  17–18, 25–29; formal, 29–32, 68; Managed Care, 6, 13, 14, 121, 140; managed
  risk contracting, 107–108; needs assessment, 38–39; paid family caretaking 13,
  109–111; standard of, 136–137, 140;
  subsidy, 10, 28, 64–66, 69; work, value
  of, 122–123, 130; work, women's, 21–22
Chichin, Eileen, 88
Christiansen, Kathryn, 13

class, 25–27
clients, 7–8; individuals 106–108; communities, 105–107
Collopy, Bart, 41
consumer-driven service models, 125–127.
  See also independent provider programs

Daniels, Norman, 151n13. See also capabilities
dementia, 83–85, 94–95, 96
dependency, 6, 7, 61–64; and dependency
  workers, 61–64, 145n13. See also Kittay,
  Eva
diagnosis-related groups (DRGs), 13–14,
  29, 31, 82
Donovan, Rebecca, 128–129
Dubler, Nancy, 80, 90

Ehrenreich, Barbara, and Deirdre English,
  21–22
elderly: ageism against, 75–76; alienation
  of, 76–78; authoritarian attitudes toward, 78–80; caretakers of, 4, 27, 76;
  dementia of, 83–85; as home care recipients, 74–75; women 4, 6–8, 74
ethics, 3, 6, 7, 54; of care, 54–56; communicative, 112–118 (see also Habermas,
  Jürgen); formal care, 29, 68; nursing, 59;
  politicizing care, 58–60

Feldman, 31, 124, 145n18
Ferguson, Ann, 139
Finch, Janet, 4–5, 21–22
Fineman, Martha, 10, 28, 64, 65, 67, 103,
  144n1, 148n20
Fiore, Robin, 45–46, 106
Foucault, Michel, 46–48, 103, 125
Frank, Arthur, 34, 40–41
Friedman, Marilyn, 96–97

gifts, 93–97; monetary, 93–95; receiving,
  95–96. See also relationships, reciprocity in

Gilligan, Carol, 55–56, 146nn3–5. *See also* ethics, of care
Graham, Hilary, 22
Grimshaw, Jean, 57

Habermas, Jürgen, 112–118, 150n12
Hobbes, Thomas, 64
Holstein, Martha, 11, 20, 25, 64
home care supervisors, 2–3, 44, 103, 147n9
Houston, Barbara, 59
Hudson, Robert, 39

identities, 138–139. *See also* Nelson, James
independent provider programs, 125, 127, 133–134, 151n4. *See also* consumer-driven service models
Ingram, David, 110, 112, 114, 150n11

insurance: health maintenance organizations (HMOs), 12–13; Medicaid, 14–16, 31, 144n3; Medicare, 14–16, 20, 31; private insurance, 16–17; risk, 107–108

Jennings, Bruce, 23
justice: for caretakers, 62–72, 84; in home care, 69–71; non-maleficence, 100–101

Kane, Rosalie, 104, 107, 144n9; and Arthur Caplan, 102; and Carrie Levin, 103, 107–108, 144n9
Kant, Immanuel, 112–113
Karner, Tracey, 44, 89
Kaye, Lenard, 36–37
Kittay, Eva, 11, 52–63, 65–68, 76, 86, 103, 132–133, 134, 143n4, 144n8, 145nn4,6, 147nn11,17, 148nn1,20, 149n1
Kuhse, Helga, 59
Kuttner, Robert, 12, 123

MacIntyre, Alasdair, 136–138, 150n6, 151n12. *See also* care, standard of
Mahowald, Mary, 63
Marxism, 121, 124; alienation of workers, 121–122
McCluskey, Martha, 64–65
medical technology, 80–83; air-fluidized beds, 81–82; catheterization, 82; feeding tubes, 82–83

Nelson, Hilde, 43, 44, 87

Nelson, James, 43, 44, 87, 138–139
Noddings, Nel, 55, 85, 95, 100

Okin, Susan Moller, 147n16
Ozar, David, and David Sokol, 33–36

Perry, Twila, 27–28
Pousada, Lidia, 81–82
Prado, Carlos, 46–47
professional roles, 36–38
profits, 38–39
public and private realm, 8, 53, 64, 89, 92, 125, 131–132, 135

race, 25, 97. *See also* Blackwell, James
racism, in clients, 97–100, 149n3
Rawls, John, 62–63
relationships, 150n9; fictive kin, 44–45, 88–89, 102, 145n5; loyalty in, 42–43; reciprocity in, 40, 94–97, 99
Roberts, Dorothy, 26. *See also* race; racism, in clients
Ruddick, Sara, 55
Ruddick, William, 81, 149n11

Schultz, Vicki, 122
Sen, Amartya, 16, 133–135, 139, 140. *See also* capabilities
Sherwin, Susan, 58–59
Silvers, Anita, 126
Stone, Robyn, and Yoshiko Yamada, 71–72
Strickling, Bonelle Lewis, 57–59

Tronto, Joan, 39, 54, 70, 145n2

unions, in home care, 7, 71, 124, 128–130, 151n6
universal health care, 123–125, 147n13; health care reform, 11–13; markets in home care, 31, 121–124; profits, 38–39

values, 33–36; in home care, 6, 33–35

Walker, Alan, 56
Walker, Margaret, 35–36
Waymack, Mark, 141–142
Wendell, Susan, 23
Williams, Oliver J., 99–100, 116

Zuckerman, Connie, 41

*Jennifer A. Parks* is Assistant Professor in the Department of Philosophy at Loyola University in Chicago. Her articles have appeared in major journals such as *Hypatia* and the *Hastings Center Report*.

DATE DUE